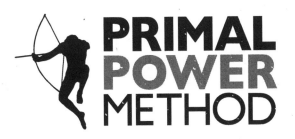

THE ORGANIC CAVEMAN

How To Make Natural And Sustainable Food Choices For Weight Loss And Health

GARY COLLINS, MS

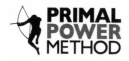

(Primal Power Method Series)

The Primal Power Method
The Organic Caveman: How To Make Natural And Sustainable
Food Choices For Weight Loss And Health
(First Edition)

Printed in the United States of America

Official program text for the Primal Power Method Series: The Primal Power Method
Copyright © 2014

Published by Second Nature Publishing, Albuquerque, NM 87109

DISCLAIMER OF WARRANTY
This material may not be appropriate for everyone, particularly for anyone
suffering from any disease or recovering from a physical injury. Any time
you intend to make a change in your nutrition or exercise program consult
with your physician for guidance and to gain clearance to participate in such
a program. The intent of this material is to further educate you in the area of
nutrition, not to diagnose, treat, or cure any physical, mental, or any other
conditions that should be under the advisement of a doctor.

Statements contained in this product have not been evaluated by the Food and
Drug Administration (FDA). None of the products or services offered in this
program are intended to diagnose, treat, cure or prevent any disease.

The text and other related materials are for informational purposes only.
The data and information contained herein are based upon information
from various published and unpublished sources that represent, health and
nutrition literature and practice summarized by the authors and publisher.
Even though the authors have been as thorough as possible in their research,
the publisher of this text makes no warranties, expressed or implied, regarding
the currency, completeness, or scientific accuracy of this information, nor does
it warrant the fitness of the information for any particular purpose. Any claims
or presentations regarding any specific products or brand names are strictly
the responsibility of the product owners or manufacturers. This summary of
information from unpublished sources, books, research journals, and articles
is not intended to replace the advice or attention of health care professionals.
It is not intended to direct their behavior or replace their independent
professional judgment.

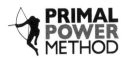

CONTENTS

About the Author

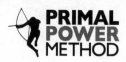

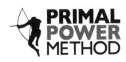

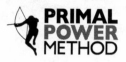

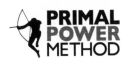

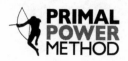

About the Author

Gary Collins, MS was born in Southern California and raised in the High Desert at the basin of the Sierra Nevada mountain range. He has been involved in organized sports, nutrition and fitness for over 30 years.

A self-declared sports junkie, he participated and excelled in various organized sports since the age of seven. He is extremely passionate about the pursuit of optimal health in mind, body and soul. Collins has two goals: To make being healthy as simple and enjoyable as possible and to give people the truth.

Collins' background is very unique and brings a much-needed perspective to today's fields of both health and nutrition. He holds an AS degree in Exercise Science, BS in Criminal Justice and a MS in Forensic Science.

After an exciting career in military intelligence Collins worked for the U.S. State Department, U.S. Department of Health and Human Services and U.S. Food and Drug Administration as a Special Agent. His career took him around the world and gave him a unique perspective on not only how the United States, but the world is affected by our food, drug and healthcare policies.

The highlights of his career took him from protecting some of the most powerful people in the world to investigations involving the biggest tainted pet food death case in the U.S. to the intricate dealings of one of the largest counterfeit prescription drug rings in the world. He has often said, "If American's really knew what was going on in the area of healthcare and nutrition in this country, they would be appalled."

It can be safely said no one in the health and fitness industry has the inside knowledge and background that Collins has. He is a hybrid of a high intensity health expert and an investigator rolled into one.

An author and college professor, Mr. Collins advises specialist and is a consultant for high-level organized sports programs and gyms. He is currently an exercise and nutrition consultant for the San Diego City College Men's Basketball team, one of the most successful Junior College sports programs in California. Some of his other clients include college football players for high profile programs, to include Purdue and Kansas State University.

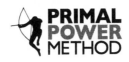

In addition to his published articles and Primal Power Method Series, he is also a contributor to the Brink of Freedom online magazine and Paleo Magazine.

Collins is a Master level personal trainer (only a few people in the world hold such a designation) with specialized training in fitness nutrition, exercise therapy, strength and conditioning, youth fitness, and senior fitness.

He is a member of the International Sports Science Association, International Mountain Bicycling Association, Nutritional Therapy Association, and the Price-Pottenger Nutrition Foundation.

Due to his unique background, Mr. Collins, conducts workshops worldwide and is a highly sought guest speaker at wellness conferences, colleges, and Fortune 500 companies.

For more information about speaking engagements or to request an interview send your inquiries to:

contact@primalpowermethod.com

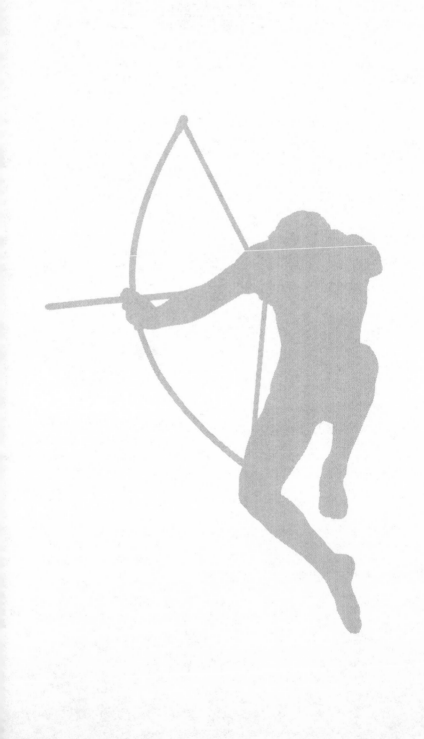

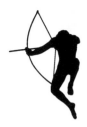

INTRODUCTION
THE ORGANIC FOUNDATION
OF PRIMAL POWER

Lasting weight loss.

All-day energy.

A lean, sexy body.

Lifelong health.

Who wouldn't want all of these?

I'm here to tell you they are all possible. You can have the body you want and the life you deserve. Even if you are starting from less than square one.

I believe it because I've lived it. And as a health and fitness professional, I have helped many people just like you achieve the high level of fitness – and more importantly, of health – that they desire. And as a former-junk-food-connoisseur-turned-healthy-eater, I've experienced it first hand.

Now it's your turn.

I believe you can lose weight and keep it off, no matter the circumstances you find yourself in today. I believe you can get off medications, improve or reverse your disease-state, and get the beach body you've always wanted, today and forever!.

But I also believe – and I know from first-hand experience – that there are a lot of forces at work trying to keep you from reaching these goals.

I'm not saying this as some crazed lover of conspiracy theories. I am saying this as a former Special Agent for the federal government and as a long-time food-industry insider. After a decade of professionally

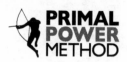

investigating the dark side of food and supplement regulations, criminal elements of the health and food industry, and the commercial marketing of Mega-Corporations who most assuredly do not have your best interests at heart, I am now here to reveal the truth.

What I Wish Every American Knew About Food

Listen, if you want to lose weight and keep it off and feel fantastic every day, you need to eat right and move your body more.

You know that already, right?

But I really need to emphasize this – there is probably nothing more important for your body's shape and your mental and physical health than the foods you eat. Almost without exception, your nutritional choices are more important than your exercise program or the vitamins you take or anything else you do health-wise.

You can summarize the effects of poor nutrition in one phrase: Garbage in, garbage out. Eat poorly, feel poorly. But the reverse is also true – eat healthfully and you can likely reverse a lot of the damage, exhaustion and weight gain that eating badly brings. My previous book and meal guide covered everything you need to know to get started on the right path in this regard.

But here's the problem – and it is a big one. The sad, sorry, and hidden truth in modern America is that if you do everything "right" with food – that is, if you go to the grocery store, buy "natural" foods including lots of vegetables and meat – you will still have substandard, problematic nutrition in your home.

Allow me to explain.

Why This Book Exists

I talk about exactly why a wholesome produce-and-meat-based diet is great for weight loss and health in my previous book, *Primal Power Method: Change Your Body. Change Your Life. The Modern Caveman Lifestyle, Simplified*. But really, it just makes sense that our bodies respond best to foods, as nature created them, doesn't it?

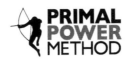

However, eating an unprocessed, whole-foods diet is so much better and more weight-loss-friendly when it's mostly or all organic. That is, foods grown the "old-fashioned" way without loads of man-made pesticides, hormones, chemicals or modifications to the genetic code of the plant involved.

Let me repeat that: I strongly believe that eating a wholesome organic selection of natural foods will benefit your health and improve your digestion relative to eating non-organic versions of the same foods. This, in turn, will boost your weight loss and health results.

Why? You are what you eat. When you eat better quality foods that mirror Mother Nature's intention as closely as possible, you will be healthier, and the weight will come off more easily. And you will feel fantastic.

That's why I wrote this book.

Organic is Better

Now you may be thinking, isn't it important to eat lots of vegetables, fruits, seeds, nuts, and animal proteins such as meat and eggs, whether or not they are organic?

In a word, yes.

Let me emphatically agree that if you eat a diet of non-organic versions of these foods, you would be way, way better off than folks eating processed junk food, greasy fast food, or the innumerable amounts of fake foods that populate the shelves of your average corporate mega-market.

That's so important, I want to repeat it: Eating a diet of minimally processed, fresh or frozen non-organic whole foods (principally consisting of fruits, vegetables, nuts, seeds, meats, poultry, eggs, and dairy products) is a far, far, far better approach than eating the stuff most Americans unfortunately do... you know, the ever-popular white breads, pastas, pastries, canned foods, pre-packaged meals, deli meats, convenience snacks, sodas, sugary mega-coffee-drinks, and pretty much any "foods" that come in a box or bag with colorful marketing images on the outside.

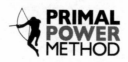

Here's the thing: Eating organic versions of natural, Primal foods will undoubtedly help you feel more energetic and lose a bit of weight, relative to the white-flour-and-sugar-driven diets most Americans consume. Organic foods are usually more expensive, but they are undoubtedly worth it.

That's the whole reason I wrote this book: You'll never achieve optimum health without understanding the benefits of organic, humanely raised, sustainably farmed whole foods.

Because even if you eat a solid non-organic diet of mostly vegetables and meat and dairy products from the supermarket, you will still be eating substandard, chemical-laced products that are only sad shadows of their organically grown counterparts.

That's what this entire book is about.

Why should you believe me?

Well, I have a few fancy academic credentials to my name, which you can read about in this book's author's bio if you want to know more. But the main reason is this: For many years, not too long ago, I worked in the Food and Drug Administration (FDA) and U.S. Department of Health and Human Services (HHS) as a Special Agent.

I've been behind the curtain of the food and supplement industry – way behind – so what I say is not based on some far-fetched conspiracy theory. I was there and witnessed it firsthand.

After a decade of federal investigations, I wanted my contribution on Earth to evolve along with my growing knowledge of the unfortunate bill of goods about food being force fed to the American public. I wanted to progress from being an investigator of the shady side of the food-and-supplement world to becoming a public health advocate. I wanted to get the information normally relegated to the proverbial back alleys of government agencies into the light of public discourse.

So, a few years ago I left my FDA job and created the Primal Power Method.

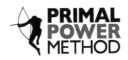

A Brief Primer on the Primal Power Method

The Primal Power Method is a concept I developed to help people make educated decisions concerning their health. The Primal Power Method website is where I share valuable free information concerning nutrition, exercise, recipes, healthy product reviews, health-related articles, special promotions and anything related to general wellbeing.

I consider my blog to be a place where like-minded "Primal Power People" can get together and chew the fat (no pun intended). I encourage my followers to share any health-related information that they think the rest of you will find useful. Remember there is no one way to optimal health, so it is always nice to learn from a new perspective.

Why is it called "Primal" power? Well, at the heart of the Primal Power Method is the so-called "Caveman" or "Hunter-Gatherer" approach to eating.

Here's what I mean by this: While we have many creature (and culinary!) comforts in our modern lives, our bodies and digestive systems have changed little since our prehistoric cousins found the secret to life-long health: active lives and natural foods.

So, we need to eat and move like they did. It doesn't get simpler than that! The secrets of health and longevity today are the same as they were thousands of years ago for our prehistoric ancestors. This idea is at the heart of the Primal Power Method.

Note that the Primal concept is somewhat similar to the popular "Paleo" diet (named after the Paleolithic period) but has several key differences. Perhaps most significantly, the Primal approach encompasses a whole-lifestyle approach, whereas most Paleo schools of thought tend to be food-centric.

None of this is to say you need to live like a caveman – far from it! Hey, I don't want to give up my car or computer either.

But when it comes to your body, realize that the diet and movement patterns that kept our species alive and empowered for many millennia

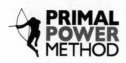

haven't changed. Anytime you are confronted by a seemingly confusing health choice, just think of how your primitive brethren would have lived... with whole natural foods and an active lifestyle. That, in essence, is Primal Power.

At the core of the Primal Power Method, is the belief it's important to strive for what is realistic rather than idealistic. We are not "food monks" and there is more to life than following a strict diet at all costs.

In this spirit, the Primal Power Method follows five truth-based, real-world principles designed to keep you on track. These form the practical foundation of the Method:

1. Knowledge is power

2. Avoid extremes

3. Keep it simple

4. Something is better than nothing

5. Take action today and every day

You can read about these concepts in detail in my previous book: *Primal Power Method: Change Your Body. Change Your Life. The Modern Caveman Lifestyle, Simplified.* Suffice to say, the whole goal of the Method is to disseminate real-world how-to tips for sustainable weight loss and good health.

To this end, the Primal Power Method advocates a realistic lifestyle, not some idealized "perfect" diet and exercise plan that nobody with a job or a family or a life has the time or energy to understand, much less follow. Adopting a Primal lifestyle can take some effort and has an initial learning curve, but once you get the hang of it, your whole family can live this way for the rest of your lives, without ever feel deprived or overwhelmed.

My previous book discusses the core of the Primal Power Method: nutrition, supplements, and exercise, including how to benefit from a balanced macronutrient intake (that is, how to eat the right amounts of carbs, fats, and proteins for optimal health and weight loss).

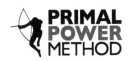

This volume is designed complement that book, and will cover the reasons you should eat organic, unadulterated versions of the kinds of wholesome foods recommended in my previous text.

It can also, however, be read as a stand-alone work for those of you seeking more information about organic foods and sustainable agricultural practices.

I believe the more information you have about why you should be doing something, the more likely you are to actually do it and to see the results you want. So we will cover a lot of information together.

In the first half of this text, we'll outline the problems facing the average American who wants to eat a healthy, natural diet. We'll discuss:

- How modern agricultural practices have strayed far from the traditional farming techniques used just several generations ago
- Why Genetically Modified foods are not all they are cracked up to be
- The horror show of modern animal husbandry that will make you want to skip the steak at dinner tonight
- The problems with pesticides and other chemicals under, on, and in non-organic foods

The second part of this book will give you the solutions to these concerns. We'll consider:

- What the term "organic" really means
- How organic foods benefit your health, the environment, and your local economy
- How you can continue to enjoy meat and dairy products while supporting humane animal faming practices
- How to navigate the confusing world of "natural" and "organic" food labels
- Where and how to buy organic and local foods
- Tips for making an organic lifestyle work with a real-world family budget

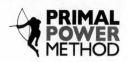

In summary, the purpose of this book is to introduce you to a new way of thinking about the foods you eat. It exists to help you eat more humanely, without supporting animal cruelty or practices that are detrimental to the environment.

I want you to eat organically, and to avoid the health-and nutrient-sapping side effects of pesticides, long-distance food transportation, and other Big Industry agricultural shenanigans that drive a company's bottom line but not a consumer's wellbeing. I want you to eat locally, supporting your farming neighbors and your regional economy. And I want you to eat real food, as found in nature, as your prehistoric ancestors did.

Unfortunately we have been brainwashed that healthy food is just too expensive, too hard to find, and just not worth the trouble. In this Primal Power Method book, we are going to dispel all those myths and get you and your family on the right track.

I will not deceive you: eating healthfully can be a little complicated at first, because a lot of the information about this lifestyle is not provided in the right format or is hard to find. That's why I created the Primal Power Method and this text.

You may have already read my other books, such as *Primal Power Method: Change Your Body. Change Your Life. The Modern Caveman Lifestyle, Simplified.* If you have, you know that I pride myself in giving you the best, most straightforward information possible. After reading this book, you will have all the information you need to find the proper organic foods right in your locale, and to improve your health and life.

In summary, it is my sincere hope that this book inspires you to experiment with (and perhaps commit to eating) better quality foods, for both you and your family. Let's get started.

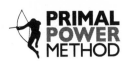

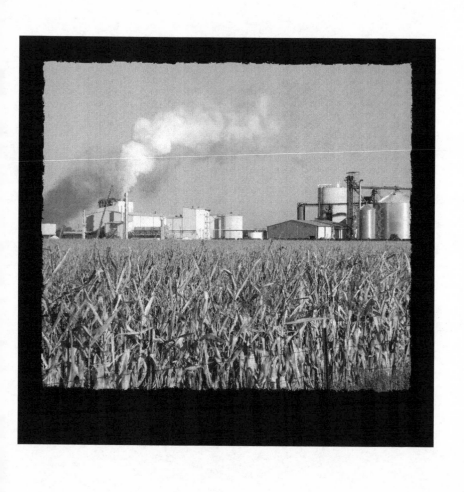

PART I
PROBLEMS

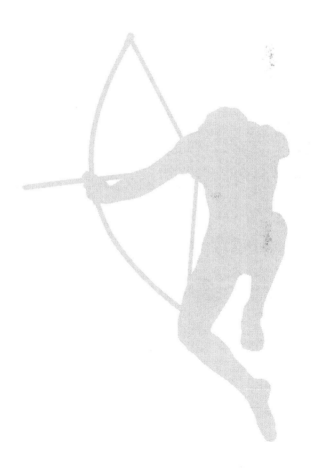

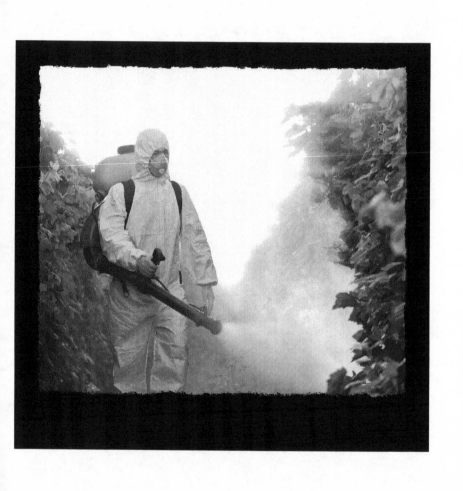

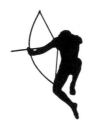

CHAPTER I
THE SAD STATE OF MODERN AGRICULTURE

Agricultural Ignorance Isn't Bliss

There has been a huge change in America that I have witnessed during my lifetime.

What is it? Americans' new and near total ignorance of, and dissociation from, the food they eat and they way it is produced.

While I was growing up (and I'm not that old, folks) everyone in my neighborhood had a small garden. Now these gardens may have only sustained a few varieties of produce such as seasonal fruit like strawberries or grapes, but they were gardens that required dedicated tending. Most of us also kept chickens; our family kept laying hens for several years.

One thing we all did have was fruit trees in our yards. I remember everyone eagerly awaiting the first batch of ripe fruits, and then the joyous neighborhood fruit exchange would begin!

I was raised in California. This great state was more widely known for its agriculture than its cosmopolitan cities a mere 50 years ago. It was in this environment that I grew up – in a small town that still maintained its ties to old-time ranching.

Today this type of localized farm heritage is pretty much unheard of.

That being said, I was not raised on a farm and would not consider myself anywhere near an expert in agriculture. But that is just it: my family members were not farmers yet we still chose to tend gardens

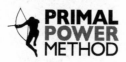

and understood their importance. Amazingly this is what we consider "organic" food today, yet it was simply the clean, homegrown produce that we once raised in our own backyards.

In the back of your mind you are probably saying to yourself, "I just don't have the space for a garden. Times have changed and a home garden today is completely impractical."

But have times really changed? I remember my grandmother's wonderful garden... behind her mobile home in the heart of Los Angeles! I still have fond memories of visiting her there.

Upon first waking every morning, she would take my sister and me out to help her tend to her fruits and vegetables. She was able to grow enough in that small area to prepare meals and even can (preserve) a little for the winter. Why? My grandmother had lived through the Great Depression, and even though she and my grandfather lived a comfortable middle class life, they never forgot how to use almost everything and they wasted very little.

For most of us in America, these time-honored traditions have radically changed. And the situation is just getting worse.

The Modern Farm: Would Your Grandmother Recognize It?

It was not that long ago when everyone either was, or knew, a farmer.

It was a simple and pivotal fact of life that one would know his or her local farmers and come to trust them, since they provided life and health through the high quality of their products. The farmers were supported in their honest, hard work by the patronage of their neighbors and friends.

This model of interdependent prosperity and abundance enlivened the members of every community where it flourished.

Even today, when I think of a farm, I think of a pleasing setting where all animals and plants live under the sun on the green earth in balance and harmony with the rest of nature. I can hear the cows mooing, chickens

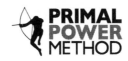

clucking, horses neighing, pigs oinking, dogs happily barking, the breeze rustling the cornstalks (non-genetically modified corn of course), and the farmer on a tractor working hard in the fields. I can smell the fruits ripening on the trees in the orchards.

Sounds pretty good doesn't it?

At least while I was growing up this is what defined the hallmarks of a typical farm.

These days, however, such a depiction couldn't be further from the truth.

Do parents even send their kids to farms for the summer anymore? Even when I was a kid this tradition was fading away, but families still did it. What better skills in life could you experience: learning how to raise your own food, butcher it, and then make it into delicious healthy meals. I consider these to be vitally important life skills – not the ability to garner 10,000 "friends" on Facebook!

Today's agricultural megalith is a far cry for the pastoral ideal of yesteryear. Indeed, were it not for the disgusting odors wafting on the breezes downwind from the average modern factory farm, most people wouldn't even know if a farm was nearby.

Simply put, my own grandmother wouldn't recognize the modern farm, and for that matter wouldn't even consider the activities of such an establishment to merit the description of "farming."

Truly, today we are facing a farming crisis.

Because Big Agriculture dominates the landscape and the popularity and knowledge of farming is at an all time low, the average age of today's farmer is 57. The U.S. has had a 30 percent increase in the number of farmers over the age of 75 and a 20 percent decrease in the number of farmers under the age of 25. As these ageing farmers retire or leave the business there currently are not enough young farmers to take their places.

And the wellbeing of our fellow countrymen is decreasing as a result.

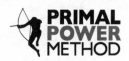

PRIMAL POWER METHOD

America's Expanding Waistlines

Now where did this disconnect between our current ways of life and the origins of our food begin? Well, I'm not exactly certain, but it has become apparent that over the last 20 years or so the American obesity epidemic has exploded.

And I believe these events are absolutely related –that's what this book is all about.

According to the international Organization for Economic Co-operation and Development's 2011 *Society at a Glance* Report:

> People in the United States spend only 30 minutes per day on average cooking, the lowest in the OECD, (which is almost half the time as other countries) as well as spending low amounts of time eating (1 hour 14 minutes per day, the third lowest in the OECD). But one third of Americans are obese, the highest rate in the OECD.

The report goes on to say:

> People in the United States have a life expectancy of 77.9 years, lower than the OECD average of 79.3 years, despite having the highest public and private spending on health at 16 percent of GDP, considerably higher than the OECD average of 9 percent.

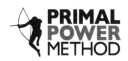

In addition, Americans spend the least amount of their disposable income on food compared to citizens of other developed countries, such as Mexico, China and Russia.

Just how little do we spend on food? According to the United States Department of Agriculture's (USDA) Economic Research Service, in 2010 Americans spent only 9.4 percent of their disposable income on food compared to 22 percent spent by Mexicans, 28 percent spent by the Chinese and 37 percent spent by Russians.

By contrast, in 1929 Americans spent almost 25 percent of their income on food; boy, how things have changed! For most of you this sharp reduction in food spending may seem to be an encouraging statistic, pointing to American dominance in the arena of world economics and the triumph of cheap food!

The USDA

The United States Department of Agriculture (USDA) is the federal executive department responsible for developing and executing U.S. federal government policies on farming, agriculture, and food.

It aims to meet the needs of farmers and ranchers, promote agricultural trade and production, work to assure food safety, protect natural resources, foster rural communities and end hunger in the United States and abroad.

Statistics, however, reveal there is more to the story.

Of the 9.4 percent of our income spent on food, almost half of those dollars are spent on meals we do not prepare for ourselves (that is, on dining out or purchasing ready-to-eat food items). Let me put this in perspective: we are spending nearly a half trillion dollars on "junk food/ fast food" per year in this country. Wow!

The fast food industry spent more than $4.2 billion on marketing and advertising in 2009, focusing extensively on television, the Internet, social media sites and mobile applications. With this kind of advertising money

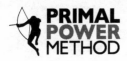

being thrown around it is no wonder that Americans are becoming more reliant on purchasing food away from home, preparing fewer meals from whole ingredients, and becoming increasingly unhealthy in the process.

Now don't get me wrong; I'm not out to close down the fast food industry.

But I remember going to fast food chains while growing up with my family as a special treat, maybe a couple times a month. We certainly didn't eat at them every single day the way so many Americans do today.

We need to take a step back and review our eating habits from a new perspective. But I believe this will be tough, because we as a society have never been so disconnected from our food sources as we are today.

America's Systemic Disconnection from Food

On September 22, 2011, *PR Newswire* released the findings of two national surveys about how agricultural products and animals are grown and raised during "The Food Dialogues," a town hall-style discussion presented by U.S. Farmers & Ranchers Alliance (USFRA). Some of the highlights of these findings were:

- 72 percent of consumers know nothing or very little about farming or ranching.
- 69 percent of consumers think about food production "at least somewhat often [sic]."
- 70 percent say purchase decisions are affected by how food is grown and raised, with nearly three-quarters (72 percent) of Americans saying they think about this topic while purchasing groceries.
- 79 percent of consumers say producing healthy choices for all consumers is very important for farmers and ranchers to consider when planning farming and ranching practices.

From the above it appears that Americans think about food quite often and think that food quality is important, yet actually know very little about where and how food is produced.

Just a hundred years ago natural farming and husbandry (the cultivation and production of edible crops or of animals for food) formed the

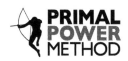

backbone of this country's economic prosperity. Food is life and producing healthy plentiful food is true prosperity! Where did it all go wrong? How did "all natural" become "genetically modified"?

A recent article in the Huffington Post noted that most children in New York City think their food comes from a grocery store. I recently watched a news program that indicated today's children didn't know strawberries came from small, ground-hugging plants. And yet we are surprised to see an eight- or nine-year-old child who weighs more than a normal, full-grown adult and who may have already started puberty, partially due to their precocious levels of body fat, and ingestion of hormones found in today's foods.

As a nation of consumers alienated from the sources of our sustenance, we have definitely lost our way.

The good news is that it appears people are starting to realize those fad-based 15-DVD exercise routines are not the answer to our weight problems, but that it mainly comes down to our dietary choices.

To find out just where our relationship with real healthy food came to an end, let's take a look at the modern factory farm and its origins.

Where Did The Modern Farm Come From?

In the film *Food, Inc.: How Industrial Food is Making Us Sicker, Fatter, and Poorer and What You Can Do About It,* journalist Eric Schlosser (himself the author of another influential book on our eating habits, *Fast Food Nation*) does a magnificent job of describing today's modern factory farm.

As a matter of fact I guarantee you that this film will have a profound effect on how you shop and what you put into your body. Probably the most notably reprehensible scene is when a farm worker is pushing a sick cow that can no longer walk with a forklift into what appears to be a slaughter pen. That is right; that sick cow likely ended up in your hamburger!

Did you also know that your industrially produced hamburger consists of meat commingled with thousands of cattle from many sources—some even from other countries—and is treated with ammonia in order to kill any bacteria and other harmful microorganisms?

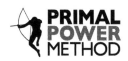

19

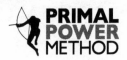

Now you see why it is becoming more difficult for the United States Department of Agriculture (USDA), Centers for Disease Control (CDC) and Food and Drug Administration (FDA) to pinpoint sources of poisonous food outbreaks. They can no longer trace an outbreak to one animal or a small group of animals, due to "Big Agriculture" (loosely translated as massive, corporatized farming interests) running our food system.

To learn how we reached this low point in national food safety, let's take a deeper look into the modern factory farm.

General consensus states that the modern age of agriculture began after World War II, as industrialized countries went back to their peacetime economies and the developing countries now free of previous dictators took control over their own food supplies.

With this came the advent of improved technology in the medical arena, such as antibiotics, and a need for peacetime markets for the many chemicals developed during the war—thus the great boom of synthetic pesticides in many forms as well as synthetic fertilizers.

In the area of agriculture farmers no longer had to work their land completely by hand. Modern machinery was developed to work the fields. This meant farmers could plant and harvest in greater magnitude than ever before.

Other modern improvements also emerged, including electric and gas stoves, refrigeration, and transportation of commodities over greater distances. Innovations such as herbicides, and heartier cultivars (plants developed through cross-breeding) initiated the trend toward reliance on single crops, rather than the old model of widely diversified farm crops.

Wheat was the first crop to be really mass-produced and signaled the beginning of carbohydrate-heavy diets as a market for vast wheat harvests.

The American Norman Borlaug played a pivotal role in developing semi-dwarf, high-yield, disease-resistant varieties of wheat in Mexico, where he established the International Maize and Wheat Improvement Center (CIMMYT) in 1964. Beginning in 1944, he spent the first 10 years breeding wheat cultivars resistant to disease and made 6,000 individual crossings.

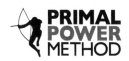

What he delivered was more wheat for less chaff (protective casings). The results? In 1943, Mexico imported half its wheat but by 1956 Borlaug had made Mexico self-sufficient, and by 1964, Mexico exported half a million tons of wheat.

It sounds great at first glance, right? I imagine that's what folks in the 1950s thought also. But after many decades of this way of thinking, the results are downright scary. Let's examine how this came to be.

Thus Began Monoculture: The Beginning of the End

As agriculture became more "sophisticated" and less traditional, farmers continued to become more and more specialized in crop production, and produced fewer and fewer varieties of crops on greater tracts of land.

It had formerly been the norm for farmers to grow several cash crops (to be sold upon harvest instead of used by the grower), as well as all the crops necessary to support the animals (and humans) on the farm.

This tradition of polyculture (raising several crops in the same space or farm) was followed for the benefit of the land and self-sufficiency, but also for a certain degree of financial insurance. If the farmer instead mainly relied on one farm product for his economic future, all it would take is a dip in the price of that product or one bad harvest and the farmer could be doomed.

Polyculture is what traditional farmers primarily practice. Polyculture is the process of raising a variety of crops and/or animals. Monoculture is raising one or a very limited number of crops and/or animals. Industrial monoculture is the dominant form of agriculture today.

To the average American, this difference in agricultural styles may not seem like such a big deal, but actually the ecological, human, and even moral effects of the hegemony of monoculture are nothing short of drastic. Here's why.

Monoculture, Monopoly, and Malaise

As the trend in monoculture increased across the U.S., the number of farmers began to shrink. Farms of thousands of acres managed by a single operator began to displace the many small, diversified farms stewarded by a tradition of family inheritance. To prop up this new

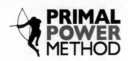

industrially scaled agricultural model and to keep cheap food flowing through the U.S. economy, the federal government instituted the subsidy system.

These industrial "farmers" would not have to worry about financial ruin because the government (actually the tax payer) would pay them to raise that crop no matter what the economic conditions. This had three unfortunate results:

1. Farmers began to leave traditional farming (polyculture) behind or left farming altogether, following the mantra of the time of "get big or get out."

2. Industrially scaled "farmers" became reliant on the government to dictate not only what they would grow, but consequently what sorts of foods would appear on grocery shelves.

3. Monoculture contributed to the rapid destruction of soil fertility via the abandonment of traditional crop rotation and increased dependence on chemical fertilizers and pesticides.

The ultimate consequences? Today's industrial monocultural farm is far more vulnerable to disease and pest problems for various reasons such as:

- Poor soil conditions due to over-farming and heavy dependence on chemical usage.
- Not having other types of crops around that naturally control pests (monocrops are susceptible to mass disease and/or insect infiltration).
- Using genetically modified seeds.
- Not using natural, locally produced compost and fertilizer from animals and plants.
- Concentrating animals in small confined areas that increase stress on the animals and thus lower immunity and invite epidemic disease (more on this later.)
- Continuous soil tilling by large industrial machinery.

These problems lead to increased usage of chemical fertilizers, pesticides, and antibiotics on farmed plants and animals, leading to short, miserable lives for these living "commodities." These practices ultimately pollute the land, the water, and the food they are producing. And the American consumer, in the unenviable position at the top of this befouled food chain, suffers greatly from disease and poor health as a direct result.

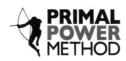

Polyculture: A Better Alternative

By contrast polyculture is the model generally in practice among smaller farm operations and organic farmers. There are many advantages to polyculture for the farmer, his crops and animals, the environment, and the consumer.

Some of the advantages to polyculture are:

- Better yields due to less soil degradation.
- Using only the best seeds from previous yields, resulting in better crops and feed for animals.
- Decreased use or elimination of herbicides, pesticides, growth hormones and antibiotics.
- Less disease due to stronger, healthier crops and animals.
- Increases local biodiversity, thus helping to maintain proper ecological balance.
- Far superior (taste, nutritional profiles of) products brought to the consumer.

One of the main reasons polyculture is not more common is it is more labor intensive to the farmer. These farms are essentially unrecognized by federal agricultural agencies and are therefore not eligible for government subsidies (should they even want them) because they just do not comply with government guidelines for eligible "farms."

Despite such narrow-minded government policies, when it comes to better food, environmental balance, and the care and happiness of the animals, polyculture wins everytime!

The Modern Grocery Store

Although this section focuses on the plight (and blight!) that is industrial agriculture, I would be remiss not to mention the confusion that exists on the other end of the food-buying spectrum: the muddling gauntlet of the average grocery market. I appreciate living in a day and age of plentiful consumer choices. But for everyday folks who want to make the healthiest choices… well, it's almost as if grocery stores were set up to confuse and bedazzle us and keep us from our weight loss goals.

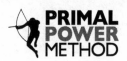

Sadly the commercially-driven, money-takes-all philosophy that dominates the psyche of modern agriculture seems to be just as prevalent in the aisles of the name-brand grocery stores and mega-markets you find in just about every town in American today.

These days, the average chain grocery store contains over 48,000 items. If you were to purchase one item per day it would take you over 131 years to buy them all!

Is it any wonder that today's consumer is confused about what to eat?

Now I hope you are thinking, why in the world does a grocery store need to carry so many items? The answer is (unsurprisingly) so the mega-food industry can make tons of money, of course. What better way to accomplish that goal than by confusing you with complicated food labels and feeding you nutrient-deficient junk to which you will soon be addicted?

Additionally, did you know there are over 320,000 food and beverage products available in the U.S.?

We are constantly bombarded with advertisements of the next miracle food, doctored to appeal to simple taste preferences via large amounts of sugar and cheap, damaged vegetable oils which provide little or no nutritional value.

It is any wonder we are facing an obesity epidemic!? It is estimated that one out of three Americans are obese and two out of three are overweight.

Our healthcare costs are ballooning along with our waistlines and are bankrupting the nation. Our entire lives are spent being hammered by food (and pharmaceutical) advertisements! All we think about is that next Big Mac and 2,000 calorie latte, both of which have virtually no nutritional value.

But they do have real value to the food giants and the healthcare system. They keep you in a constant state of hunger and sickness. But don't worry. With the Primal Power Method (and, frankly, common sense) we are going to stop this unhealthy roller coaster and educate you on how to navigate that grocery store and all its enticing items.

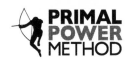

When I consult or talk with people the key health-boosting skills most do not have is a knowledge of how to shop for and select healthy foods, and also the basic skills to prepare these foods.

I'm astonished that most Americans have no idea how to shop intelligently for food, not a clue. To make matters worse, if they have to turn on that thing with four burners in the kitchen, a fire is more likely to result than breakfast, lunch, or supper. As a matter of fact you should have seen the look on my own mother's face when I told her, "You need to learn how to cook to get your health in order!" I honestly thought I might see tears. Yes, people, just because I live a healthy lifestyle does not mean I come from a family of health gurus. They fight all the same battles you do.

Even for me, navigating the average supermarket is confusing.

First, it takes me forever to find anything, considering there are 48,000 items to search through.

Second, if I need to find a healthy food item, which is an almost impossible feat in these types of establishments, reading the product label hurts my head. Yes, even those pesky food labels can confuse me at times as well. Okay, it doesn't contain any GMO products, but does it have high fructose corn syrup? Wait, is that soy I see at the bottom of the list, and what does "flavor enhancing" mean?

It goes on and on. To be honest, I just try to avoid those massive grocery stores since it is nearly impossible to shop and eat healthfully at these places.

That is why the much smaller and more health-conscious stores such as Trader Joe's and small local specialty markets are gaining in popularity. They have far fewer items and are probably a tenth of the size of the mega-supermarkets.

The funny thing is, when I suggest that someone patronize one of these smaller stores to help improve their shopping and eating habits, I often receive the response, "I don't like those stores as they don't have very many options."

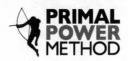

Who needs an entire aisle, tens of feet long, that only offers sugary soft drinks and chips? No matter what chain grocery store you go to you will always see that same aisle. It makes you realize quickly who has the most influence over your food choices. Let me give you a hint; it's not you!

Do you ever wonder why almost every large chain grocery store's inventory is laid out identically? A lot of time and money was spent on research to make sure you go where they want you to go and buy what they want you to buy.

I'm here to tell you those massive grocery stores are designed for you to buy the most nutrient-empty products possible. Why do you think all the real foods—such as fresh fruits, vegetables, and meat—are on the outside walls of the store and all the items you shouldn't be eating are in the center? Why do you think all the candy is right there by the cash register?

Marketing research has shown that if you stare at it long enough while waiting your turn in line, you are very likely to buy it on impulse, even if you managed to avoid it in the treacherous center aisles. If you manage to avoid purchasing the candy at the register I guarantee your kids— whose impulse control is weaker than an adult's—will not!

The interesting thing is these big chain grocery stores are catching on that people want more organic and healthy options and are starting to carry more of these items. Of course they make sure to lead you through stack of decidedly unhealthy items even during your quest for quality choices.

Recently I was on an extended trip and I was picking up some organic staples from Raley's grocery store chain because someone had told me they now have an entire section dedicated to organics. That fact was partially true.

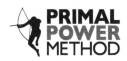

PRIMAL POWER METHOD

When It's Available, People Choose Health

An article published in the *Journal of Preventative Medicine* found positive and statistically significant correlations at both the community and the zip code level between the availability of healthful products in stores and the reported healthfulness of individual diets.

In other words, if healthy foods are locally available, more people will buy them and use them. And, by extension, the community will be healthier. Isn't that the kind of place you'd like to live?

When I walked in the front doors there was no clear indication where these healthy items might be located, so I had to wander through those dangerous center aisles packed with food pretenders in tempting colorful plastic packaging until I finally found the so-called "organic section."

Still, the healthful food selection was not entirely clear to the customer; it was split into several parts. There was one section devoted to refrigerated and frozen organics, and then dry goods were located in the next aisle. These organic items were mixed in with foods that I would not recommend or consider healthy. The organic fresh produce required me to navigate to yet another part of the store where again they were mixed with GMO and conventional produce.

Clarifying the Terms "Conventional" and "Traditional"

Note that by "conventional" foods, I mean non-organically grown foods, i.e. those grown using agri-industrial and modern technologies, such as synthetic pesticides, inhumane husbandry practices, and so on.

When I about write "traditional" farming techniques, I mean the kinds of methods your great-grandparents would have used (i.e., organic before the term organic was invented!).

I will use these semantic references throughout this text.

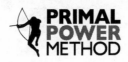

All right; I know when I'm being duped. I have spent nearly half my life studying and working in the field of criminal investigations so I can recognize tricky marketing when I see it. By satisfying your desire to have more organic choices, they have still made sure you get to see less healthy foods along the way for ultimate temptation.

When I later took my mother to Raley's for her to purchase some organic items that is when it truly all came together. My mom (who represents the average customer well as she is not "into" holistic living) was completely confused and could not distinguish the healthy items from the ones that were not.

Yes, this is how they want it; you may come in for that half gallon of organic milk, but what good does it do you when you are eating it with the supposed "health" cereal Cheerios that you bought because of a slick marketing plan? Those of you who follow the Primal Power Method will know that all cold breakfast cereals are nutrient-empty slurries of junk and are in no way healthy. (See page 139 of this book for more.)

I believe Marion Nestlé puts it best in her book *What to Eat*. Here she describes the dynamics and the seedy relationship between the mega-food industry and massive grocery store chains.

> This unsavory system puts retail food stores in firm control of the marketplace. They make the decisions about which products to sell and, therefore, which products you buy. This system goes beyond [the] simple matter of supply and demand. The stores create demand by putting some products where you cannot miss them. These are often "junk" foods full of cheap, shelf-stable ingredients like hydrogenated oils and corn sweeteners, made and promoted by giant food companies that can afford slotting fees, trade allowances, and advertising [i.e. different types of fees paid to grocery stores by the producers of food to have their products placed in the most visible locations in the store, be favorably promoted, etc.].

> This is why entire aisles of prime supermarket real estate are devoted to soft drinks, salty snacks, and sweetened breakfast cereal, and why you can always find candy next to the cash register. Any new product that comes into a store must come with guaranteed advertising, coupons, discounts, slotting fees, and other such incentives.

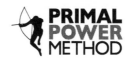

Basically these chain supermarkets seem to give you what you want on the surface, but what good does it do if you still are confused and are unable to make healthier choices?

You are probably asking yourself why I dedicated such a great deal of discussion on the modern grocery store? The bottom line is I consider the modern grocery store ground zero for America's health epidemic. This is where over 90 percent of the population gets its food, so for me it's something that deserves a great deal of critical attention.

After not regularly shopping in these stores for years, when I step into a modern mega-supermarket today it is very obvious to me why people are confused about food choices and their health. I know I was once one of those people. I shopped at these stores for many years, and was fooled into purchasing items that I thought were healthy. Today shopping for food has become incredibly difficult and confusing for the average American and I hope you can learn from my experience and mistakes.

We will explore how to avoid these chain supermarket pitfalls later in this book. Once you understand how to shop for the proper health-giving foods, safeguarding and optimizing your health and wellness become much easier.

For now, let's revisit an issue that has a huge impact on the choices you need to make at the grocery store and on how Big Agriculture is poised to totally dominate food growing in our country. I am referring, of course, to genetically modified foods.

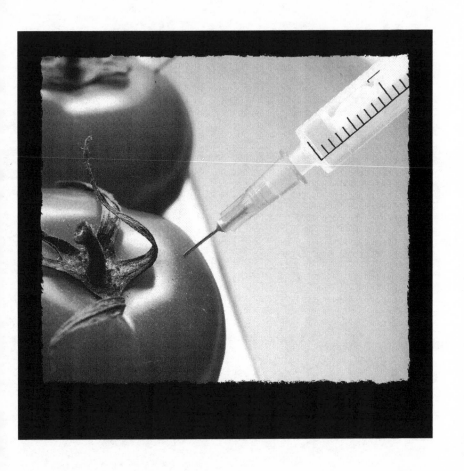

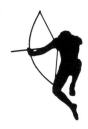

CHAPTER 2
GENETICALLY MODIFIED FOODS

What are GMOs?

A huge reason to choose organic foods is that they are not allowed to be genetically modified.

That is a simple statement. Yet this is such a big topic I have given it its own section in this book, so you may adequately understand why GMO foods should be avoided in your diet.

GMO stands for *genetically modified organism*, which refers to any food product that has been altered at the level of the working subunits of an organisms DNA "blueprints," or genes. Genetically modified foods are also frequently described as genetically engineered, genetically altered or genetically manipulated (a.k.a. GE, GM, or GMO.)

Of course for hundreds of years farmers crossbred their plants to favor preferable characteristics, but crossbreeding is far different from the process GMO crops undergo. Essentially in GMO, the genes of a crop are turned on/off, removed or altered by a technician in a laboratory, in an attempt to make the plant more resistant to pests or chemicals used during the pesticide spraying process.

Sound good? It may be... or it may be deadly. No one really knows for certain. The main concern when it comes to consumer health is that scientists are unsure of how these genetic manipulations will affect our short- or long-term health.

We are barely scratching the surface when it comes to understanding how agricultural genetics work and how they affect human beings or the animals we feed these products to.

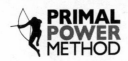

We are just beginning to understand that our DNA can be damaged or made healthy by what we consume in the form of food. It was once thought our DNA was static (it didn't change), but we now understand that it can be greatly affected by environmental factors, including what we eat. To make matters worse these changes in our gene expression, caused by poor nutrition or GMO's, can be passed on to our offspring.

Are you willing to take that gamble with your own health – or your children's?

A Growing Controversy

Genetically modified or engineered food (GM or GMO) has become a hot topic of conversation over the last few years. Indeed as I have worked on this book, there has been a huge push for the FDA to require food labels on any product containing genetically modified ingredients.

As a matter of fact, on March 27, 2012 a record-breaking goal of one million signatures in favor of GMO labeling was reached, which is more signatures than any other food petition previously submitted to the FDA. More than 40 countries worldwide, including all of Europe, already have GMO labeling.

You have probably seen an article or news program on the issue recently, but you may not understand what all the fuss is about. So here's the deal.

Most people don't understand that GMO food products are big money. Over the last 10 years, the agriculture biotech industry has spent over a half billion dollars in lobbying to make sure the consumer is kept in the dark.

GMO crops became commercially available in the United States in 1996 and currently constitute the vast majority of corn, cotton and soybean crops grown in the country. More recently, biotechnology firms have developed genetically engineered animals, including food animals like hogs and salmon. Today, some estimates indicate that over 90 percent of all soy and corn grown in the U.S. is from genetically modified seeds.

Here's why you should care.

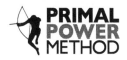

Why Are GMO Foods Considered Detrimental to Our Health?

Research on the effects of GMO products on health is where the meat of the controversy lies.

There is now a large amount of evidence that toxins in certain GMO foods may trigger inflammatory responses, food allergies, and cause infertility.

Take the case of GMO tomatoes. To create one, tomato genes are spliced with a fish gene in order to make the tomato frost-resistant. The result is people with fish allergies could have a reaction to the tomato or even die from eating such a manipulated tomato.

Recent animal studies showed genetically modified foods caused the following detrimental health consequences:

- Lung damage
- Stimulates immune response (the body's reaction to possibly harmful foreign substances)
- Lower birth rates
- Higher mortality rates of offspring
- Inability to reproduce

Mad Cows?

According to Organic Authority June 21, 2012, what's being called "mysterious cattle deaths" in Hesse, Germany, has led to criminal charges filed against Switzerland-based multinational biotech company, Syngenta, for allegedly covering up animals' deaths recorded in trials that resulted from the ingestion of the company's genetically modified Bt176 corn variety. Farmer Gottfried Gloeckner filed the charges after losing a civil lawsuit in 2007 against Syngenta for the loss of some of his herd between 2000 and 2002.

In addition, researchers linked glyphosate (the active ingredient in Roundup weed killer) to Sudden Death Syndrome (SDS), a serious plant disease, in many fields around the world. Numerous studies have shown

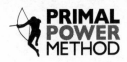

that glyphosate contributes not only to the huge increase in SDS, but also to the outbreak of some 40 different plant and crop diseases. Glyphosate weakens plants and promotes disease in a number of ways, including the following:

- Acting as a chelator (a particular way that ions and molecules bind metal ions) of vital nutrients, depriving plants of the nutrients necessary for healthy plant function
- Destroying beneficial soil organisms that suppress disease-causing organisms and help plants absorb nutrients
- Interfering with photosynthesis, reducing water use efficiency, shortening root systems and causing plants to release sugars, which changes soil pH
- Stunting and weakening plant growth

So why are they even made? Well of course it's easy to think that GMOs are easier to grow and may therefore be cheaper and more abundant for us to consume. But even this is an unsatisfactory argument, as you are about to discover.

Do GMO Crops Have Any Benefits?

Supporters of GMO food believe that this technology makes it possible to produce enough food for everyone to have enough to eat. This is supposedly accomplished by making sturdier and more pest-resistant crops. But while GMO crops may be cheaper at the supermarket checkout line, the cost to our health (and burden on our healthcare system) is, in my estimation, incalculable.

Agriculture biotech companies have also promised drought-resistant and high yielding, genetically engineered seed, but that has yet to come to fruition.

Unfortunately, the agriculture biotech companies who create these products almost always produce or support all of the positive research regarding the "benefits" of GMO crops. Talk about the fox guarding the hen house!

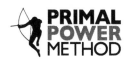

We have already mentioned the potential health problems associated with GMO crops and products, but GMO products also cause environmental problems. Instead of creating crops resistant to weeds, which is one of the biggest benefits claimed by the agriculture biotech industry, the opposite is produced: a new breed of super-weed that is immune to the herbicides used for weed control.

Now instead of using less herbicide, farmers use more and more herbicide to battle these garden nuisances. Not only does this cause the foods we eat to contain higher levels of these chemicals, but those chemicals also seep into the soil and ground water, contaminating our environment.

Studies also find that rather than producing more crops when using GMO seeds, farm production is actually decreasing, especially when compared to farmers using polyculture and sustainable farming techniques.

Not only are the GMO farmers doing far more harm to the earth than their small sustainable farmer counterparts, but they also have lower output and higher costs to raise their crops and animals.

One factor most people do not know is that, through the lobbying of special interest groups, these biotech companies have made it illegal to replant the seeds produced by their GMO plants. Thus the farmer must purchase new GMO seeds every year adding to the bottom line of farmers.

This is especially tragic for farmers in Third World countries, the very population these companies tout that they are helping. These farmers are now held hostage to these multi-billion dollar companies, all in the name of greed.

Yet instead of producing better yields, and weed and pest resistant crops, the very opposite is happening. Rather than helping feed the world these companies are actually helping to starve and steal from them. I know these words may seem harsh, but the truth often has some sharp barbs attached to it.

I'd like you to steer as clear of GMOs as you can. Eating organic foods will help you do that. So will becoming aware of what foods are typically genetically engineered.

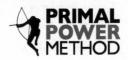

Common GMO Foods

Here is a partial list of everyday foods that are typically genetically modified (source: Butcher, 2009): honey, soybeans, tomatoes, corn, sweet corn, canola, potatoes, papayas, cotton seed oil, meat and dairy products, (i.e., meat and dairy animals are often fed GMO feed), peas, vegetable oil, and sugar beets.

But it's not just "normal" foods that are genetically altered. Here is a list of some of the ingredients, additives, and flavor-modifiers that are frequently added to processed foods. You may not even know what a lot of these are. Well, as a general rule I recommend you don't eat anything you can't pronounce or that sounds like a chemical accident about to happen.

The fact that these are commonly genetically modified is just one more reason to always read food labels and avoid anything that contains these ingredients. Just eat real food!

- Aspartame (Also Called Aminosweet, Nutrasweet and Equal)
- Canola Oil (Rapeseed Oil)
- Cellulose
- Citric Acid
- Cobalamin (Vitamin B12)
- Colorose
- Condensed Milk
- Confectioners Sugar
- Corn Flour
- Corn Meal
- Corn Oil
- Corn Sugar
- Corn Syrup
- Cornstarch
- Cottonseed Oil
- Leucine
- Lysine
- Malitol
- Malt
- Malt Syrup
- Malt Extract
- Maltodextrin
- Dextrose
- Diglyceride
- Fructose (All)
- Glutamate
- Glycerides
- Glycerin
- Glycerol
- Glycine
- High Fructose Corn Syrup (HFCS)
- Hydrogenated Starch
- Hydrolyzed Vegetable Protein
- Inverse Syrup
- Inverted Sugar
- Isoflavones
- Lactic Acid
- Sorbitol
- Soy Flour
- Soy Isolates
- Soy Lecithin
- Soy Milk
- Soy Oil
- Soy Protein

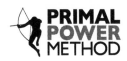

- Maltose
- Mannitol
- Milk Powder
- Milo Starch
- Modified Food Starch
- Mono And Diglycerides
- Monosodium Glutamate (MSG)
- Nutrasweet
- Oleic Acid
- Phenylalanine
- Phytic Acid
- Protein Isolate
- Vegetable Fat
- Vegetable Oil
- Whey
- Whey Powder
- Xanthan Gum
- Soy Protein Isolate
- Soy Sauce
- Starch
- Stearic Acid
- Table Sugar
- Tamari
- Tempeh
- Teriyaki Marinades
- Textured Vegetable Protein
- Tocopherols (Vitamin E)
- Tofu
- Triglyceride

Natural Does Not Mean GMO-Free!

Sadly, there are thousands of products that are not certified as non-GMO, but are GMO nonetheless.

For example, in 2011 the Cornucopia Institute tested several "natural" labeled products, and the results were startling! They found numerous "natural" products, such as the ones listed below, contained high levels of GE ingredients, sometimes as high as 100%:

- Kashi (GoLean)
- Mother's (Bumpers)
- Nutritious Living (Hi-Lo)
- General Mills (Kix)

For non-organic, "natural" products making "non-GMO" claims, results showed that these claims cannot always be trusted.

Barbara's Bakery (Puffins) and **Whole Foods' 365 (Corn Flakes)**, which are both enrolled in the Non-GMO Project, contained more than 50% GE corn.

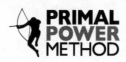

Kashi – and most especially their **GoLean** product line – has taken a great deal of heat lately for misleading the consumer. Their products were labeled 100% Natural, and it was found by the Cornucopia Institute that some of them contained 100% GMO grains and several chemical additives.

This is why I always tell people to remove cereals and breakfast bars from their diet. Not only are they more likely to have GMO grains, they are also filled with sugar, chemicals, and processed white flour. I explore these topics much further in my other Primal Power Method resources, available on my website www.PrimalPowerMethod.com.

How to Avoid GMO Products

As you can see, product labels can be very misleading and confusing when it comes to choosing GMO-free items. So what should you do?

The easiest way to avoid GM products is to purchase items with the "100% USDA Organic" sticker on the label.

Federal law requires that organic food products be produced in a manner that promotes ecological sustainability, without the toxic inputs and genetically engineered ingredients common in the conventional food system.

One of the best ways to get GMO-free fruits and vegetables is to belong to a Community Supported Agriculture (CSA) group or buy your food from a local farmer or Farmer's Market. Of course you have to do your research when buying from a local farmer to make sure they follow proper organic practices.

We will expand on the above points later in this book.

The bottom line: The best way to avoid GMO products is to buy "USDA 100% Organic" foods. However, this advice might one day change as companies are devising ways to get around this.

Some estimates say as many as 30,000 different products on grocery store shelves are "modified." That's largely because many processed foods contain soy. Half of North America's soy crop is genetically engineered!

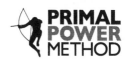

A good resource for GMO info is the Non-GMO Project's website: http://www.nongmoproject.org. The Non-GMO Project is a non-profit organization committed to preserving and building sources of non-GMO products, educating consumers, and providing verified non-GMO choices. You can search their website to find non-GMO products and retailers who only carry non-GMO products.

The Non-GMO Project is an incredible free resource and I highly recommend you add them to your arsenal of health and wellness info.

Hopefully you will now have some better tools to recognize and avoid GM foods and products. Always pay attention to labels, and remember if you find them confusing, it's for a reason: to make it harder for you to decipher a good product from a bad product. When in doubt, just don't eat it.

Genetically Modified Vitamins?

Remember vitamins and supplements can also contain GMO ingredients, so you will have to pay attention in this area if you use these products.

Vitamin C (ascorbic acid) tablets are often made from corn, and vitamin E is usually made from soy (a majority of all corn and soy grown in the U.S. is GMO). Vitamins A, B_2, B_6, and B_{12} may be derived from GMO's as well as vitamin D and vitamin K may have "carriers" derived from GM corn sources, such as starch, glucose, and maltodextrin.

Beyond the Concerns of GMOs

Some last words of wisdom when it comes to GMOs: Just because a product is listed as a confirmed non-GMO product it doesn't necessarily mean it is good for you. Those of you who have read my previous book *(Primal Power Method: Change Your Body. Change Your Life. The Modern Caveman Lifestyle, Simplified)* will remember that what's most important is the quality of the foods you eat.

Remember: A non-GMO certified cookie is nevertheless still a cookie!

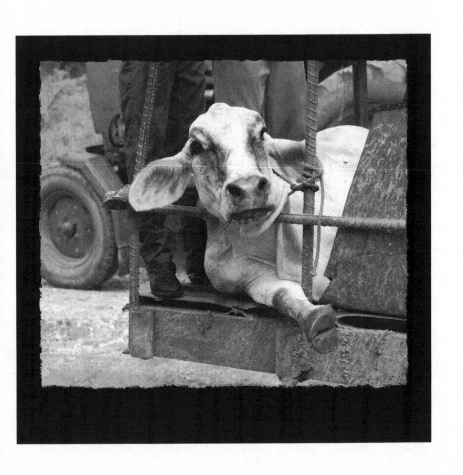

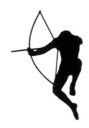

CHAPTER 3
ANIMAL CRUELTY FOR THE SAKE
OF STEAK

The way we raise, slaughter and process animals for consumption in America is nothing short of atrocious. It's yet another "dirty little secret" that the food mega-corporations prefer you do not know.

But let me be ultra-clear about the importance of meat: I don't want you to be a vegetarian.

I prefer that you to include animal products – meat, poultry, dairy, eggs, and sometimes fish – in your menu plans. However, the problems with non-organically raised animals are so all-encompassing, and exist on so many levels, they deserve their own section in this book.

(Incidentally, if you want to know more about health issues related to vegetarianism, meat and protein consumption, and why I so adamantly recommend including animal products in your diet, check out my previous book: *Primal Power Method: Change Your Body. Change Your Life. The Modern Caveman Lifestyle, Simplified.*)

Here's why you should make an extra effort to include organic animals in your diet… and the awful consequences that can occur when you don't.

The Meat We Eat

It is estimated there are over 100 million cattle in this country at any given time. We slaughter 35 million of them each year, resulting in 26 billion pounds of meat. Each year about 8 billion chickens get turned into 43 billion pounds of chicken products. Lastly there are 96 million pigs slaughtered and a few million lambs.

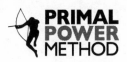

Would it surprise you to know after seeing these numbers that only a very small number of very large companies are responsible for all this meat?

Indeed, it's a sad truth that only a small handful of companies produce the majority of our meat and poultry products. For example, only four meat processing plants slaughter approximately 80 percent of all beef and 50 percent of hogs in the U.S. And did you know that Tyson Foods alone owns 25 percent of the country's meat supply?

This is not good folks – Mother Nature is not a fan of stifling diversity, and we have definitely tinkered with her plans on this one.

Now, I'm no anti-capitalist or anywhere even close. However, when it comes to food production and you have a very small number of very large, powerful players aided and abetted by the federal government, then it is guaranteed that bad things are going to happen to the consumer.

Meat is big business and I will tell you the mega-producers do not want you or your small organic farmer getting in their way. These food companies spend billions of dollars every year in advertising and government lobbying to make sure they determine what you will eat.

You may be thinking that all of this has nothing to do with you. That's where you are wrong.

These big food industries are literally making us sicker by the national hegemony of their mass food raising and processing techniques. Do you know how hard it is to track down the source of contaminated meat when they are slaughtering tens of thousands of animals per day? Remember I used to work for the FDA, so for me, this question is not just academic.

Let me tell you, it is virtually impossible. And when a company wields that kind of power do you think the consumer is ever going to be protected? I think not; and as a matter of fact I know not. Remember, I was there, on the inside.

And here are the terrible details about this industry that insider's know.

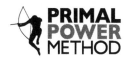

Concentrated Animal Feeding Operations (CAFOs)

As modern commercial agriculture and farming have taken over, disastrous husbandry techniques have been concurrently developed.

Today's "animal farms" are pumping out tens of thousands of pounds of meat daily. In order to maximize profits and meet this kind of market demand, the **concentrated animal feeding operation** (CAFO) was born.

Think of a pastoral, family farm, where livestock graze happily on fresh grass and calves nuzzle happily at their mother's side as they grow under sunny skies. Now imagine the polar opposite of this idealized, small family farm situation and you come close to the reality of the modern CAFO.

A CAFO is essentially a massive animal factory designed to produce as much meat or poultry with as few natural resources as possible. In this set up, huge amounts animals are kept for at least a couple of months in vegetation-free, industrial-type settings. It's not nice.

For anyone who has seen a true CAFO operation... well, to say it is frightening is a gross understatement. I have no idea how these operations avoid the consequences of animal cruelty laws. If anyone were to treat their family pet in the way a CAFO treats its animals he or she would surely be turned in by their neighbor and arrested.

Below is a sampling of some typical treatments of animals condemned to spend their short, miserable lives in CAFOs.

- Their entire lives are spent in dark, crowded conditions wallowing in their own excrement and urine, and with the overpowering stench these conditions produce.

- Chickens' beaks and claws are clipped to prevent pecking or scratching each other to death because of the stress induced by their unnaturally confined conditions.

- Pigs have their teeth and tails removed because when tightly confined they tend to gnaw other pigs' tails near them as a high stress response.

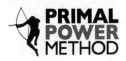

- Mass slaughtering of smaller animals may be attempted via large voltages of electricity that will not kill all the animals the first time administered, causing great suffering and terror.

- Animals are fed cheap GMO rations that are foreign to their digestive systems causing disease and sickness for most of their short lives.

- Hormones and large doses of antibiotics are administered to unnaturally fatten the animals in order to bring them to market sooner. Some chickens have also been bred to grow so fast and produce so much breast meat that they become abnormally top-heavy and their legs are not strong enough to hold them upright.

- An estimated two-thirds of all U.S. cattle raised for slaughter are injected with growth hormones.

- Some of the things animals are fed in CAFOs: same-species meat, other diseased animals, feathers, hair, skin, hooves, blood, manure and other animal waste and plastics.

- In the U.S., approximately 95 percent of egg-laying hens (that's around 300 million) are confined to tiny cages stacked several high in dark warehouses. This is the only life they will ever know.

It's just common sense that, if you want to be healthy, these are not the kinds of animals you want ending up on your dinner plate. You are what you eat!

Choose healthy, happy animals (organic meats) to ensure your food dollars support humane husbandry techniques, and to ensure the food you serve your family is the healthiest selection possible.

Animal Cruelty

Some might say that killing and eating animals in any way is the ultimate manifestation of animal cruelty. I must say that I disagree.

As previously noted, I discuss my stance on vegetarianism in greater detail in my previous book, *Primal Power Method: Change Your Body.*

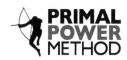

Change Your Life. The Modern Caveman Lifestyle, Simplified. But suffice to say I do encourage you to eat humanely raised or wild organic meats, fish, and poultry; the natural cycle of life means that many animals must consume other animals in order to survive.

The right kind of meat, however, does not include the products of CAFOs. Remember that modern agriculture and these animal mega-farms are very recent phenomena in human civilization.

Here's the bottom line: The practices used today in a modern CAFO are deeply disturbing and I believe if people truly knew how the animals they were eating were treated, you would see an overnight boom in the popularity of small farms that embrace traditional (humane) husbandry techniques.

Allowing an animal to experience a life of pain and suffering in a CAFO just because in the end it will just end up in your stomach is not a reasonable excuse for the inhumane practices of these "animal factories." But it's easy to disregard the conditions in which your food is raised when you only see the end product in plastic-wrapped packages that are ready to eat.

Environmental Impact of CAFOs

CAFO's create moral and nutritional dilemmas, certainly. However, their damaging reach is not confined to the animals they house nor the consumers they "nourish." Sadly, CAFOs also are a blight on the earth and very damaging to the environment.

A major reason for this is that, since by design they purposefully confine thousands of animals in the least amount of space, CAFOs produce an incredible amount of animal and chemical waste.

Not only are the animals exposed to this waste, but the farmers and their employees—not to mention all neighbors downwind and downstream—are also exposed to these deleterious waste products as well.

In order to deal with this amount of animal feces, CAFO operators dump it into large, stagnant lagoons or dry-spray it onto open land. Eventually this toxic dump ends up in our drinking water when it is absorbed by the ground or washed away in rainwater.

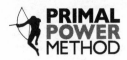

PRIMAL POWER METHOD

Large farming operations will usually mix low doses of antibiotics with the feed and water in order to make livestock grow faster and attempt to fight the many diseases that arise from such crowded and unnatural conditions.

According to the Union of Concerned Scientists, seventy percent of all antimicrobials used in the U.S. are used on livestock. This is more than twenty-five million pounds of antibiotics a year, or eight times what humans are administered yearly!

We now know the detrimental effects of using large amounts of antibiotics: super-organisms that have developed resistance to the very chemicals meant to annihilate them. The Europeans have understood the self-destructive perils of this dangerous behavior, and the agricultural use of antibiotics is banned in many countries, with a resulting decline in these sickness-causing super-organisms.

> **Unnatural Husbandry = Unnatural Disease Conditions**
>
> A study published in 2004 in the *Journal of Occupational and Environmental Hygiene* examined the possibility that inhalation of microorganisms could be a health concern for workers inside and downwind of animal confinement units (i.e. animal mega-farms).
>
> Researchers found that disease-resistant bacterial forms were found inside and downwind of the swine confinement facilities, indicating that resistant organisms were being produced in and released from these facilities. Resistance to a battery of antibiotics including ampicillin, erythromycin, oxytetracycline, penicillin, tetracycline and tylosin was found.

Disease on Your Dinner Plate?

What happens when you concentrate thousands of animals in a small space, feed them substandard or species-inappropriate foods, and force them to breathe the stench of their own feces and urine?

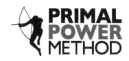

Disease happens.

Almost every outbreak of human disease can be attributed to humans or animals being confined in overcrowded unsanitary conditions.

Think about it. If you concentrate a group of animals in an enclosed, tightly confined area, what would Mother Nature have to say about this arrangement? Mother Nature would think these animals have overpopulated a geographic locale that was not meant to support that number of animals.

The easiest way to weed out the weak and reduce the numbers of animals and thereby reduce the stress in that environment would naturally be via the mechanism of disease. This latter stance is my opinion and not based on scientific readings, but it does seem like a common sense conclusion.

The bottom line here is that Mother Nature knows a lot more than we do when it comes to matters of ecologic harmony and balance. And since we are ultimately a part of nature, I believe we mess with nature at our peril.

CAFOs and Disease

The Journal of Vector-Borne and Zoonotic Diseases indicates influenza pandemics occur when a novel influenza strain, often of animal origin, becomes transmissible to humans. Domestic animal species such as poultry or swine in concentrated animal feeding operations (CAFOs) could serve as local amplifiers for such new strains of influenza.

"Mad cow" disease is a prime example of how mass animal production stifles health.

In order to save money, farmers often use feed derived from other animal parts. Scientist believe mad cow disease is spread when cattle are fed tissue from the nervous system(s) of other cattle, such as the brain and spinal cord of other infected animals. Now, I'm not a biochemist or molecular biologist, but even I know feeding sick animals to other animals is a really bad idea.

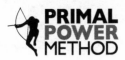

The Chicken Loophole

According to the U.S. Food and Drug Administration:

> As the regulator of animal feed, [the] FDA plays a key role in protecting U.S. cattle from bovine spongiform encephalopathy (BSE), also called "mad cow" disease, and protecting the health of people who consume cattle products. In April 2008, FDA issued a final regulation barring certain cattle materials from all animal feed, including pet food. The banned materials are the cattle tissues that have the highest risk for carrying the agent thought to cause BSE. The final regulation strengthens a 1997 feed regulation and subsequent amendments to protect animals and consumers against BSE.

So how do our ever-creative industrial agriculture friends decide to fix the problem? Instead of feeding cows the grisly dregs from the cattle slaughterhouse, they decided to feed them ground up chickens. Honestly people, I can't make this up.

But there is only one problem with this brilliant solution: there are still (possibly contaminated) bovine remnants in the ground up chicken meal.

That's right, chicken litter, a cooked and rendered mix of chicken manure, dead chickens, feathers, and spilled feed, are all marketed as cheap feed rations for cattle. The beef industry likes it because this mess is cheaper than even GMO corn and soy.

It is estimated that two million pounds of chicken litter are fed to feedlot cattle each year. (Mmmm, just ponder that appetizing fact the next time you savor your non-organic, feedlot burger!) But here's that problem we were referring to earlier. It is estimated that about one-third of the chicken litter mix is spilled feed, which just happens to include beef remnants and bone meal often used to feed chickens, but which is supposed to be off limits for cattle.

You have to love these guys. As if the GMO corn and soy weren't cheap enough to save a few production pennies they come up with the chicken litter feeding solution.

Is it starting to sink in that the mega-food industry really could not care less about the consumer? Their bottom line is entirely driven by greed.

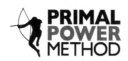

Who in their right mind would put their customers at extraordinary health risk in order to save a couple of pennies? Well, I think we know.

As far as I'm concerned such tactics are completely unethical at the very least, and in fact lean more toward the realm of criminal activity. Of course that's a view filtered through my decade as a special investigator for the FDA and U.S Department of Health and Human Services. In my experience in this capacity, I can say that if there's a legal or technical loophole to be found, someone who wants to make a few quick bucks will find it.

When I talk about being an insider in the industry this is exactly what I'm talking about. The general public has no idea what is going on with their food production. If I hadn't worked for the FDA I probably wouldn't have a clue either. But that is where they want you: dumb and in the dark.

Once the populace is educated and finally protests against their venal practices they will be forced to change their business model, which would of course compromise their bottom line. The industry just can't have that. Money, money, money!

The End Result

When you raise thousands of animals in tightly confined areas devoid of sunlight (one of nature's most powerful antimicrobial agents) and feed them inappropriate foods, drugs, and expose them to toxic chemicals, poisonous air, and other horrific treatment, bad things are simply bound to arise.

Combine that set-up with mass slaughtering practices in which thousands of animals' fluids and waste are commingled and I'm surprised we have not been hit with even worse public health outcomes. But again we would be the last ones to find out.

Most meat you find in your grocery store today comes from CAFO production. Here are just a few final appalling statistics about the modern day CAFO:

- Most animals raised for food in the United States are raised on factory farms.

- For years, investigations have revealed conditions on some factory farms that result in extreme animal suffering.

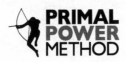

- The total number of livestock on the largest factory farms rose by more than one-fifth between 2002 and 2007.

- The average size of hog factory farms increased by 42 percent over a decade. Seven states average more than 10,000 hogs per factory farm.

- The average size of egg operations has grown by half over the last decade. The five states with the largest flocks all average at least 750,000 hens per factory farm.

- Although the EPA is tasked with regulating factory farms, it has done little or nothing to control the environmental damage caused by factory farms.

Farmed versus Wild Caught Fish

I wish I could end this discussion here. But unfortunately, meat-producing animals and poultry and not the only ones being adulterated thanks to unhealthy new farming techniques. Fish are also being subjected to tactics that increase production yet decrease health.

Industrial fish farming, or aquaculture, is the fastest growing form of food production in the world, according to FishWatch.com. About half of the world's seafood now comes from fish farms, including in the US, and this is expected to increase.

In 2011 global farmed fish production topped beef production, and the gap widened in 2012 when 66 million tons of farmed fish were produced, compared to 63 million tons of beef.

With the continued pollution of our oceans and waterways, farmed fish sounds like a great idea in theory but, just like CAFO-raised animals, farmed fish face detrimental health perils. These include pollution, receiving antibiotics, being fed GMO-derived feed, and disease.

On top of this, it has been reported recently that most fish products are purposefully mislabeled to dupe the consumer into buying a substandard product at premium prices. I have also experienced this phenomenon in my investigations with the FDA.

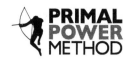

There is no easy answer to this dilemma. Healthy fish can be a wonderful, if not essential part of a well-rounded and healthful diet. What I have done myself is only purchase and consume seafood labeled "Alaskan" because it cannot have been farmed. Alaska goes to incredible lengths to protect their seafood brand and image integrity and ensure its quality and sustainability.

Another way I avoid the perils of farmed fish is to catch it myself. That way I'm guaranteed to know the source. But even that is not a perfect system, as farmed fish are planted into our streams and lakes to maintain populations.

I remember as a youngster touring the "Fish Hatchery" in the area I grew up in, as part of a school field trip. These fish were raised in order to restock the streams and lakes in the area I grew up in, the Sierra Nevada Mountain Range. Of course, I had no idea this is what was done in my area until I toured the "Fish Hatchery." I'm sure it's not exactly what Mother Nature had in mind.

So where does that leave us? I have personally greatly reduced my fish consumption, because there is just no simple remedy to this problem. It's a sad reality. But this is but a small example of the damage we are causing to our environment. The truth is that how we are raise our food directly impacts our food choices and therefore our wellbeing.

Modern Meat: Genuine Food or Science Experiment?

For those of us who are very health conscious individuals, the modern farm animal is not welcome anywhere near our plate. When you consider the numerous recent outbreaks of E. coli bacteria and mad cow disease, and bouts of stomach and lower GI issues that many people experience, modern meat is definitely something to avoid.

Marion Nestlé in her book *What to Eat* writes:

> In the mid-1990's, the USDA issued regulations that required meatpacking companies to institute safety plans and to test for hazardous bacteria. But these rules, relentlessly opposed by meat producers and processors, ended up with gaps, disincentives, and loopholes. [...]

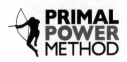

Never mind that the meat you eat might be loaded with bad bacteria. It is your responsibility to deal with the problem. Look carefully at any package of meat in the United States and you will find a "Safe Handling" label that explains the problem, although in print so small that it may need eye-glasses to read it:

This product was prepared from "inspected and passed" meat and/or poultry. Some food products may contain bacteria that could cause illness if the product is mishandled or cooked improperly. For your protection, follow the safe handling instructions.

- [Refrigerator] Keep refrigerated or frozen. Thaw in refrigerator or microwave.

- [Faucet] Keep raw meat and poultry separate from other foods. Wash working surfaces (including cutting boards), utensils, and hands after touching raw meat or poultry.

- [Frying Pan] Keep hot foods hot.

- [Thermometer] Refrigerator leftovers immediately or discard. Cook thoroughly.

Wow! Are we preparing a meal or are we preparing some kind of ultra sterile science experiment? I'm pretty sure our not-so-distant ancestors didn't worry about mixing raw meat with vegetables or sterilizing their cutting surfaces.

But this is where our modern meat raising and processing system has brought us. You now know why food irradiation (zapping meat with doses of radiation) was born: why prevent the problem of tainted meat when you can just nuke it and not worry about it?

Nice fix, I must (sarcastically) say. Obviously from the continued outbreaks of *E.coli* and other illnesses this so-called logical approach is not working. Why is that?

The simplistic approach to food safety fails miserably because animals on CAFO and mass-production farms are not only fed species-inappropriate diets, but drugs, heavy doses of antibiotics, and are exposed to a whole host of toxic chemicals in their feed and environment.

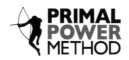

Are we surprised that many foreign countries will not allow imports of some American meat products and some have banned them outright?

But it's not just American meat that is suspect. There is one additional food group of animal origin I'd like to discuss – dairy products.

The Plight of Modern Milk

If you choose to eat or drink dairy products, it is especially important to choose organic options. Here's why.

Today's over-processed pasteurized milk options are a far cry from what your great-grandparents would have recognized or consumed.

Your body may be able to tolerate and thrive on natural, raw dairy products, but react badly to the stuff proffered at the supermarket. To understand why, we must revisit the source of the problem: the sad story of modern farm-raised cattle.The modern milk cow is a freak of nature. Just a century ago, a cow produced two to three gallons of milk per day. Today's dairy cows produce up to four times this amount.

This extraordinary output is the result of unnatural, high-protein diets and selective breeding that favors cows with abnormally active pituitary glands (the glands that produce milk-stimulating hormones and growth hormones). The controversial use of bovine growth hormones also helps to create more milk-productive cows.

The dire trade off, however, is that these unnatural hormones, which destroy the health of the dairy cow, are also passed to us through the processed milk.

This comes at great cost. Excessive pituitary hormones are associated with tumor formation, so it's not surprising that some studies have linked milk consumption to cancer. On top of this, the modern cow is prone to many diseases due to its poor diet and needs frequent doses of antibiotics to stay alive during its short life. These antibiotics also find their way into the milk supply – and thus your body – every time you drink milk from cows treated with such medications.

The quality of modern dairy products has been further compromised by the use of high-protein soybean meal as cow feed. Soy stimulates

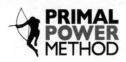

the production of large quantities of milk, but also causes a high rate of mastitis (i.e., udder inflammation typically caused by infection), sterility, liver problems and decreased longevity in cows.

Since whatever an animal eats is stored in their muscle and fat tissues, we can reasonably assume that whatever they eat, we are effectively consuming in turn. Sadly, high-protein soy feed for livestock is becoming increasingly popular and is cheaper than feeding cattle what they should naturally consume: grass.

The meat from the animals fed a soy-based diet often comes with the seemingly-healthy label of "vegetarian fed."

However that moniker can be very misleading, since many consumers naïve to the dangers of soy may mistakenly assume the term "vegetarian fed" automatically makes the meat product a healthier choice. The best selection? Look for meat and dairy products from "grass fed" animals instead. (We'll discuss these distinctions in detail in the next section.)

Food for Thought

There is a huge difference between the modern CAFO-raised animal and a happy, free-range grazing or pecking animal.

As we have seen the modern farm is a place of darkness, drugs, and cruelty. As you can imagine the same problems humans face with poor nutritional choices, high stress, pollution, and lack of exercise also apply to the animals we eat.

Common sense indicates that an unhealthy animal is not going to give the same level of nutritious food product as a happy, thriving, healthy animal – in other words, an organically-raised animal.

But before we get to the good news about how an organic lifestyle can heal the wrongs outlined in this book so far, I want to pause for a moment to share some thoughts on the food industry crises as discussed so far.

When most people are confronted full force by the insanity of conventional factory farming—whether in the shape of gruesome animal concentration camps (CAFOs) or vast, chemically dependent and

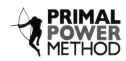

genetically manipulated "Franken-crops"—they tend to agree that kinder, healthier ways of agriculture ought to be encouraged.

When the inescapable reality of conventional agriculture is thrust under their noses, most are instinctively repelled by the gross exploitation of plants, animals, and nature in general that is the repulsive hallmark of most of this model of agriculture today. Yet many of us may not be aware that we hold considerable power in helping make that change toward healthy agriculture happen.

A perhaps uncomfortable truth is that the fractured food system we have right now exists because, as a whole, we all wanted it. We wanted cheap and plentiful food, available year round regardless of season or proximity to our door, and in as convenient a form as possible. We didn't care how that food was manufactured, how the environment that produced it was degraded, whether or not local economies perished as a result, or how much packaging and fossil fuel for trucking was wasted.

In the very same way, we, as a whole, can step into our individual power and one by one reject this model and embrace another that is healthy and holistic. Each individual can make a powerful statement simply by refusing to purchase foods produced via conventional agriculture and choosing only organic variants—especially those in season in their geographical locale—instead.

The decision to choose only organic, locally produced food is a commitment to social change as well—a decision to support and honor the larger family of all life on this planet.

Unsustainable agriculture simply means a model of farming that cannot survive without artificial props and supports. A certain number of years can go by and this propped-up model outwardly seems to function all right, but then things begin to crumble around the edges.

Serious imminent disasters such as the Colony Collapse Disorder affecting bee populations in this country and parts of Europe provide an excellent example. There are many theories offered to explain the widespread die-off of honey bees, including pesticide use, deadly pollen produced by genetically modified food crops, the introduction of new, neuro-disruptive pesticides that confound the bees' homing abilities, and the exploitation and weakening of bees by transporting them around the country to pollinate vast monocrop farms.

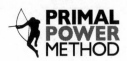

This last example may be something that most people are completely unaware of. The California almond crop, for example, is a vast monoculture of only almond trees for miles and miles. The trees blossom for only three weeks a year and native bees long ago moved on, since they of course need diversified forage in the form of pollen and nectar for the whole year, not just three weeks.

So, the almond industry must arrange to have bee hives trucked in from around the country for that blossom period in order for the trees to set fruit. This means that bees from the eastern part of the country—who are normally in a resting stage in the hive at this time—must be disturbed from badly need rest, rudely shipped across the country on transport trucks, and exposed to other transient bee populations and whatever illnesses they may have in their new work location.

This mercenary exploitation of a benevolent, selfless, and ever-giving animal is yet another shocking testimony to the heartless impulses driving conventional agriculture every day. (For more on the honey bee crisis and what you can do to help, visit www.spikenardfarm.org.)

Another example of the tolling bell of doom for conventional and unsustainable agriculture has played out in deadly heat and drought of the summer of 2012 in the Midwest. Conventional monocrops such as corn and soybeans have shriveled in hundred- and thousand-acre fields, soil has cracked in wide fissures, and even trees began to die.

Many farmers were forced to feed hay to cattle at a time when pasture grazing is usually assured. However, those small, diversified farms with a harmonious number of animals in relation to pasture acreage did not have to supplement with hay. These animals managed to find enough forage even as the many weeks of high temperatures and no rain mounted.

When the drought finally broke and abundant rain finally relieved the long drought, the diversified grass farmers saw their pastures quickly rebound with fast growing new grass. They did not suffer erosion of topsoil as did the monocrop farmers and they and their livestock emerged stronger because of the summer's trials.

This resilience in the face of adversity is a gold-standard mark of true health and sustainability. We want to see that resilience in a strong and healthy individual, and most certainly in the model of farming that we depend upon for our own health.

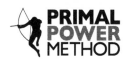

So here's the solution: Each of us must make the effort to educate ourselves as much as possible about the sources of all the foods we eat.

This commitment is a small sacrifice to make—or perhaps I could better say is a noble sacrifice to make—in order to bring about healthy changes in our agriculture and reduce the suffering it causes to so many, including those of us who fall ill because of shoddy food.

Learning where your food comes from, who grows it and how, and supporting those worthy sources is deeply satisfying and will improve not only your physical health, but, if I may say, comfort your soul.

Voluntarily choosing foods that are not only organically grown, but perhaps even more important, are seasonal to your locale is a powerful act that supports truly sustainable farming practices. Take the process on as a long-term educational project—the learning is actually very pleasurable, the people you meet along the way will be new friends and allies, and your life will become immeasurably enriched as a direct result.

All of us truly long for this meaningful interaction of community, for the soul-satisfying feeling of working together and supporting each other for the common good, as an expression of love.

Solving the Problems

The preceding discussion probably made you seriously consider becoming a vegetarian. However, that's not what I recommend – there is a better way.

Let's face it, Americans like meat and we eat a lot of it! As followers of the Primal Power Method know, I'm a proponent of getting your complete protein in the form of animal products, mainly meat.

The good news is you can and should be eating animal meat, eggs, and sometimes, dairy products. This next part of this book will reveal how to do it the right way.

So at long last, let's talk about solutions.

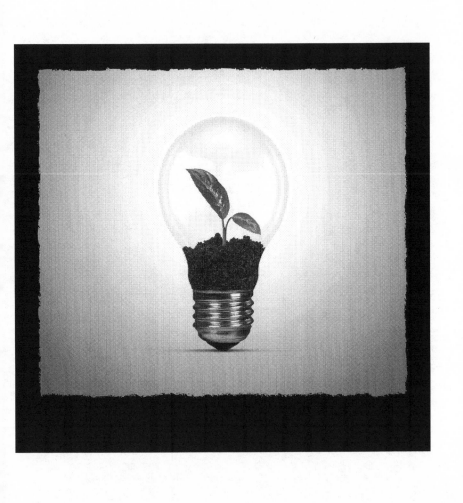

PART 2
SOLUTIONS

Consumer food choices can truly seem overwhelming when staring down the travesties that are modern agriculture, aquaculture and animal husbandry. But there is good news.

A small but vocal minority of health advocates have helped to slowly eke out legal definitions that help protect consumers from the reach of Big Agriculture and the mega-food industry. It is possible to eat well, and to avoid the pitfalls of non-organic foods. Oh, and to lose weight, look sexy and feel fantastic along the way.

Perhaps the most user-friendly of these steps forward is the legitimization of an "official" definition of organic foods, so that consumers can really know what they are buying.

So what does the term "organic" actually (and legally) mean?

Put into simple terms: organic produce and other ingredients (such as organic spices) are grown without the use of pesticides, synthetic fertilizers, sewage sludge, genetically modified organisms or ionizing radiation. Animals that produce organic meat, poultry, eggs and dairy products are not fed or injected with antibiotics or growth hormones.

This section will describe more about what make organic foods distinct from non-organic foods. We'll examine the impact of pesticides on our wellbeing, and discuss how organic growing techniques produce hardier crops. We survey the specific benefits of food products derived from organically-raised animals. And, we'll discuss how savvy shoppers can navigate the confusing world of food labels and supermarket aisles to ensure they are getting the best possible food value for their hard earned dollars.

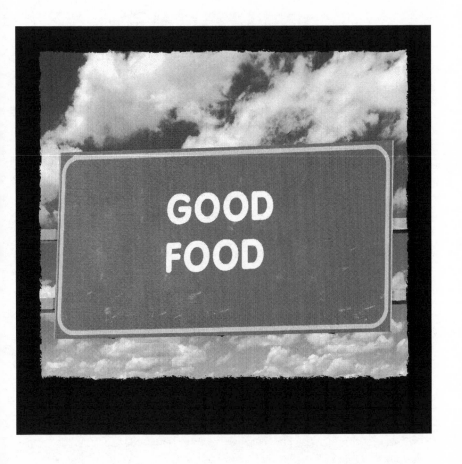

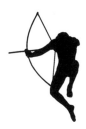

CHAPTER 4
ALL ABOUT ORGANIC FOODS

Why You Should Go Organic

Eating organic foods is better for your health, your neighbors, and the environment. In broad strokes, here are just a few of the ways organic foods help us all.

These are the benefits of organic farming to consumers:

- Certain plants cultivated in an organic system contain higher levels of health-boosting antioxidants.

- Children who consume organic diets have reduced exposure to organophosphorus pesticides, as measured by urine concentration in dietary crossover studies.

- Research demonstrates improved flavor in organic versus conventionally produced strawberries, and improved taste in organic versus conventionally produced apples.

These are some benefits of organic farming to the environment:

- An organic food production system creates healthy soils, the foundation for healthy crops.

- Farming practices in an organic system include growing diverse crops and a crop rotation plan using cover crops (plants beneficial in preventing soil erosion, enhancing soil fertility, and disrupting weed, pest, and disease cycles).

- An organic food production system eliminates synthetic fertilizers, thereby reducing nitrogen and phosphorus contamination of groundwater.

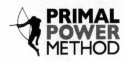
PRIMAL
POWER
METHOD

- An organic food production system conserves fossil-fuel energy.

- An organic food production system reduces the use of pesticides that persist in the environment.

These are a few benefits of organic farming for farmers:

- There are economic savings though the use of on-farm inputs, such as crop rotations and composting.

- Organically produced foods contain fewer pesticide residues.

- Farm laborers and family members benefit from reduced pesticide exposure. Exposure to conventional pesticides can have negative effects on both female and male fertility.

- In developing countries, organic farming improves community and household food security.

- Sustainable prices for organic products help farmers reinvest in their operations, and encourage young people to enter farming.

Information concerning what makes organic food items better than conventional, frequently cheaper items can get a little confusing. I hope the picture I have drawn for you above is making it clearer, but for those of you who still aren't convinced, let's compare organic and non-organic foods head to head - specifically, regarding pesticides, taste, nutrient levels, and crop yields.

Fewer Pesticides: Better for You and Better for the Planet

Probably the most important reason for you to switch to organic products, and especially fruits and vegetables, is the fact synthetic (unnatural) chemical pesticides are not allowed to be used on organic crops.

According to the U.S. Environmental Protection Agency (EPA) a pesticide is any substance or mixture of substances intended for preventing, destroying, repelling, or mitigating any pest.

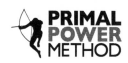

Though frequently misunderstood as referring only to insecticides, the term pesticide may also apply to herbicides, fungicides, and various other substances. Under United States law, a pesticide is also any substance or mixture of constituents intended for use as a plant regulator, defoliant (intended to remove leaves), or desiccant (a drying-out substance).

Note that "organic" plants may be treated with natural, "biological" pesticides (i.e., biopesticides) derived from animals, plants, bacteria, and certain minerals sources. The EPA notes on its website, for example, that canola oil and baking soda have pesticidal applications and are considered biopesticides. I don't know about you but I'd rather eat a vegetable from a plant treated with baking soda than sprayed with chemicals from a laboratory.

Several health risks have been associated with exposure to certain man-made pesticides. These include cancer (particularly of the brain and prostate), birth defects, spontaneous abortion, premature birth, gestational diabetes, insulin resistance, obesity, type 2 diabetes, and neurodevelopmental disorders (learning disabilities).

Have you ever eaten a piece of conventionally grown fruit without washing it first? That bitter taste that is a combination of the pesticides and herbicides used during the growing process, and perhaps a "protective" coating applied to the fruit as it was sent on transport as well.

Every time I have been unable for whatever reason to wash a conventional piece of fruit before eating it, soon after, a vicious stomachache and headache ensue. Now think of doing this everyday of your life; surely there will be health consequences for regularly ingesting these chemicals. Even if you wash these items with soap and water there will still be residue left behind.

All I do with my organic fruits and vegetables is rinse them off with plain water. In my own garden I don't even do that most of the time as I eat them right off the vine or stem.

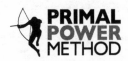

A Brief History and Some Scary Statistics

Pesticides are not a modern invention.

Elemental sulfur was used by ancient Sumerians to protect their crops from insects. Medieval farmers and scientists experimented with chemicals ranging from arsenic to lead on common crops. Nineteenth century research focused on more natural techniques involving compounds made with the roots of tropical vegetables and chrysanthemums.

In 1939, Dichloro-diphenyl-trichloroethane, or DDT was discovered to be extremely effective and rapidly became the most widely used insecticide in the world. Twenty years later, serious concerns about the human safety and biological impacts of DDT led 86 countries to ban its use.

A growth in pesticide use began after World War II with the introduction of DDT, BHC, aldrin, dieldrin and endrin, all of which are now classed as persistent organic pollutants (POPs). DDT was especially favored for its broad-spectrum activity against insect pests of agriculture and human health, such as mosquitoes.

But there was collateral damage: Under constant chemical pressure, some pests became genetically resistant to pesticides, non-target plants and animals were harmed, and pesticide residues appeared in all areas, even those not related to agriculture.

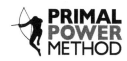

Persistent Organic Pollutants (POPs) are characterized by a long "half-life" (i.e., taking a long time to bio-degrade), by their potential to be carried over great distances by water or air, and by their capacity to build up in dangerous levels in the food chain; POPs are widely found in flora and fauna, and consequently in humans. Some POPs can cause adverse reproductive, developmental, immunological, hormonal, and carcinogenic effects in humans and flora and fauna.

According to the EPA world pesticide expenditures totaled more than $35.8 billion in 2006 and more than $39.4 billion in 2007. Expenditures on herbicides accounted for the largest portion of total expenditures (approximately 40 percent), followed by expenditures on insecticides, fungicides, and other pesticides, respectively. Total expenditures increased in 2007 due to increased spending on all pesticide types.

U.S. pesticide expenditures totaled $11.8 billion in 2006 and $12.5 billion in 2007, in proportions similar to those of world expenditures, with a relatively larger proportion of total U.S. expenditures on herbicides. In 2007, U.S. expenditures accounted for 32 percent of total world expenditures on pesticides, 38 percent of world expenditures on herbicides, 39 percent of world expenditures on insecticides, 15 percent of world expenditures on fungicides, and 25 percent of world expenditures on other pesticides.

Today, more than 20,000 pesticides are registered with the Environmental Protection Agency (EPA) resulting in a multibillion-dollar industry in the United States alone.

As you can see we are dumping and spraying tons of insecticides every year in the U.S. and it is big business. I like to call it the Agriculture Industrial Complex, because there is a network of big corporations all interdependent on each other and at the head, the U.S Government. Where do all these chemicals end up? On and in our foods, the soil, and eventually in every one of us!

The Taste Test

For decades I have seen news and television programs comparing the organic and non-organic foods, usually in a blind taste test, to show that people cannot tell the difference between organic and conventional products by taste.

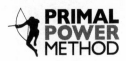

Years back I was one of those people who scanned the organic section at the grocery store, saw the prices and just kept on going. I'm sure seeing those news programs and specials were firmly planted at the back of my mind.

I would bet big money on the fact that the mega-food industry was probably behind some of these programs and specials. The good news is the organic food prices are becoming increasingly competitive versus conventional food prices.

But I will admit when it comes to taste, it is often hard to tell the difference between organic and non-organic products. With that being said I can tell the difference in certain products, especially fruit, and I can definitely taste the pesticide residue on the conventionally grown products.

In my previous writings I have discussed how modern, commercially produced food, mainly in the form of sugar and white flour, dull our sense of taste. So is it any wonder that most folks cannot tell the difference in taste between organic and conventional foods?

But when it comes to the real differences between organic and conventional food, taste variations are usually the most difficult to discern. I do notice a difference in textures and taste in grass-fed animal meat, and most people who have changed to an all, or mainly, organic diet will agree with this observation.

Of course, there are other considerations. Taste is important, but in the big picture the fact that most organic products taste similarly to conventional (non-organic) foods is far from the most important reason you should be eating more healthfully.

With this being said, know that as you detoxify your body and you greatly reduce your sugar and refined white flour consumption, your palate will become more discerning. (I discuss the dangers of sugar- and white flour-laden products in my previous Primal Power books and reports.)

Once that happens, I guarantee you will notice a difference in taste between organic versus conventional foods. It took me years to fine-tune my body (a continuing lifelong process) in order for me to tell the difference.

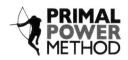

More Chemicals, Higher Yields, Less Nutrients = A Fatter You!

"Ounce for ounce, today's high-yield crops are less nutritious and deliver fewer nutrients per serving and calories consumed," notes a 2007 report from The Organic Center entitled "Still No Free Lunch: Nutrient levels in U.S. food supply eroded by pursuit of high yields."

Think about it: less nutrition, for the same calories. Not so great!

The report continues:

> For example, there have been double digit percentage declines of iron, calcium, selenium and other vital nutrients in many contemporary, high-yield crops compared to older varieties and/or lower-yielding fields. In general, the higher the yield of wheat, corn and soybeans, the lower the protein and oil content.

> High tomato yields come with lower levels of vitamin C and the cancer-fighting compounds lycopene and betacarotene. Higher levels of production on livestock farms have also resulted in erosion of nutrient density. For example, the average amount of milk produced by a dairy cow has quadrupled in the last century to roughly 22,000 pounds today. But this milk is less concentrated with fat and protein.

How Fewer Nutrients in Conventional Foods Affect Your Waistline

According to the Organic Center in Boulder, CO, a large body of research shows that organically grown foods contain more nutrients (on average, from a marginal percentage to more than 20% of certain minerals and 30% or more of antioxidants) compared with foods grown by conventional agricultural practices.

You may be thinking that it's no big deal if you get 20 to 30 percent fewer nutrients in your conventionally grown food; it is still cheaper than organics.

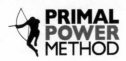

Here's the problem: in order for you to get the equivalent nutrition from non-organic foods you now have to eat at least 20 to 30 percent more of the foods than if you were to eat organically grown and raised products. This means you will now be consuming far more calories to maintain basic health and wellness. But this will probably not be good for your waistline.

This behavior is in direct conflict with the proper health and wellness model. You cannot lose weight and maintain health by eating more calories than you need in order to receive sufficient nutrition from your food.

Simply put, Americans are already consuming far too many empty calories in the form of sugar and processed foods. Add to that more calories needed to maintain basic health requirements and we have the perfect storm for weight gain, obesity, chronic illness, and a multitude of health problems.

Health-giving organic foods are typically already lower in calories than highly processed foods, thus making them waist-slimming in their natural forms.

Take into account organic foods also do not contain the chemical bath typically drenching the modern industrial food supply and you are on the road to a slim and healthy lifestyle!

When it comes to health organic is always best. In the long run and in terms of health costs and food costs, eating organic foods are actually far cheaper than eating their conventional counterparts.

> The *Journal of Alternative and Complementary Medicine* reviewed multiple studies and found that organic crops usually contained more vitamin C, iron, magnesium, and phosphorus, and significantly fewer nitrates, than conventional crops.

The Question of Crop Yields

We are often bludgeoned with the notion, delivered as obvious truth, that we cannot feed the world with that old tired organic way of farming.

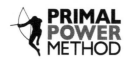

We are told we need modern, chemically-derived fertilizers and pesticides to make sure people don't starve.

To me this sounds like typical Big Industry propaganda, but what is the real story? Is it possible to feed our ever-growing world's population through self-sustaining, organic farming?

And why should we (or any one nation or consortium of nations) be so arrogant to want to feed the world when the world has always fed itself, community by community, all over this green globe?

Let's take a look at the facts and make our minds up for ourselves.

Various studies find that, compared to conventionally grown agriculture, organic crops yielded 91 percent, or 95-100 percent total crop output, along with 50 percent lower expenditure on fertilizer and energy, and 97 percent less pesticides. Stated simply, this means that organic crops yielded slightly less actual food but used way, way less fertilizer, energy, and pesticides to do so.

A 2007 study compiling research from 293 different comparisons into a single study to assess the overall efficiency of the two agricultural systems has concluded that:

> ...organic methods could produce enough food on a global per capita basis to sustain the current human population, and potentially an even larger population, without increasing the agricultural land base.

> (Source: Badgley et al., 2007)

Converted farms (farms that have converted to an organic model from a non-organic approach) have lower pre-harvest yields than their conventional counterparts in developed countries (92 percent) but higher yields than their low-intensity counterparts in developing countries (132 percent). This is due to relatively lower adoption of fertilizers and pesticides in the developing world compared to the intensive farming of the developed world.

Here's the bottom line: There are many factors that go into yields, but long term the organic approach out-produces the chemical mass-produced farms.

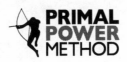

Organic farms withstand severe weather conditions better than conventional farms, sometimes yielding 70-90 percent more than conventional farms during droughts. Organic farms are more profitable in the drier states of the United States, likely due to their superior drought performance.

Organic farms survive hurricane damage much better, retaining 20 to 40 percent more topsoil and smaller economic losses at highly significant levels, compared with their non-organically grown neighbors.

Michael Pollan in a 2008 *New York Times* article, hit the nail on the head:

> In fact, well-designed polyculture systems, incorporating not just grains but vegetables and animals, can produce more food per acre than conventional monocultures, and food of a much higher nutritional value.
>
> But this kind of farming is complicated and needs many more hands on the land to make it work. Farming without fossil fuels — performing complex rotations of plants and animals and managing pests without petrochemicals — is labor intensive and takes more skill than merely 'driving and spraying,' which is how corn-belt farmers describe what they do for a living.

The bottom line reveals that the "higher yields argument" put forth by the proponents of conventional agriculture just doesn't hold water.

Big industrial farms do not have to follow the same practices as the organic farmer in the ways in which they dispose of waste, use chemical additives, and go about packaging foods and/or slaughtering animals, etc.

Their processes are not based on quality or yields like they would have us believe. Instead, their incentives are based on price per unit, or maximum return for the lowest level of resources and effort. High yields are just a benefit, but when you compare apples to apples (no pun intended) it just isn't the same.

Organic farmers do not house their animals in small confined areas wallowing in their own feces, feed them some cheap, foreign diet they were never intended to eat, get huge subsidies from the government. Organic farmers are also subject to more frequent official inspections, relative to non-organic farmers.

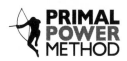

When you throw out all the special and economic privileges that conventional factory farms benefit from you will see a big difference in total output when compared to the traditional self-sustaining farmer. The self-sustaining farmer uses almost all needed resources with very little waste and that, my friends, is what healthy living is all about.

A health-supporting farming model is also a moral system that seeks to honor nature and respect animals. This is a far cry from manipulating and exploiting animal life in order to extract every last penny from each "production unit."

I don't know about you, but I sure like to sleep at night. Choosing a moral approach to my meal choices that supports positive, traditional animal husbandry techniques really helps in that regard.

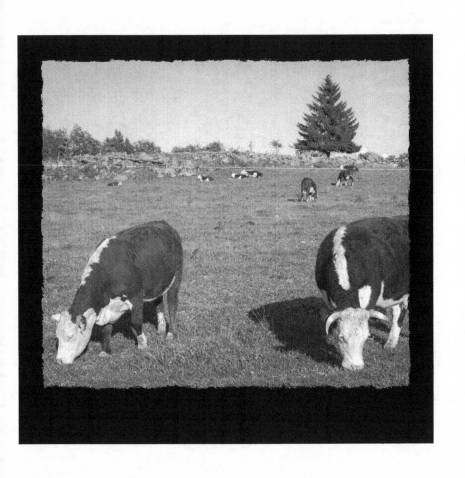

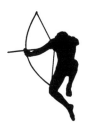

CHAPTER 5
ORGANIC ANIMAL PRODUCTS

I'm sure you have witnessed the rise in labels claiming "free range" and "grass fed" becoming more prevalent in your grocery store or local market. The American public is starting to catch on that healthy animals means healthier people, but is it worth it to plunk down the extra cash for these newly touted animal products?

My answer is an emphatic yes!

Eating the meat of an animal who has been raised in harmony with Mother Nature – outdoors, in the sunshine, close to its mother, eating the food its stomach was designed to digest, with lots of physical activity (playing, running freely) as it grows up – this is a totally different situation than the horrors of a CAFO. It's different environmentally, morally, ethically and in terms of nutrition.

Think of it this way: if you were to take your kids on a fun visit to a farm, which one would you rather go to – a pastoral, traditional family farm with happy animals… or a CAFO? It's just common sense which animal should end up on your dinner plate too.

A Grass Fed Cow is a Healthy Cow

Products from grass fed bovines are better. Why?

Here's the bottom line: Cows are not designed to eat grains, corn, and soy as their principal ration, if at all. This type of CAFO-driven diet makes them sick and is why cows on large-scale, commercial farms usually require large doses of antibiotics to suppress their symptoms of poor health.

Cows are designed to eat grass, period. The rumen (the largest compartment of a cow's four-part stomach) is where ingested grass is broken down by bacteria that naturally live in the cow's gut.

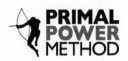

These same bacteria are not, however, efficient at breaking down the grains, corn, and soy products that the modern cow consumes today. The grains also alter the pH (acid/base balance) of the bovine rumen, preventing normal digestive function.

Making matters worse, the corn and soy that is fed to most commercially farmed cows is nearly always genetically modified (GMO). You will recall from our earlier discussions that GMO products are highly controversial and generally considered to be unhealthy.

This is a major reason why **free-range, grass-fed beef** and organic dairy products are becoming increasingly popular. Remember: You are what you eat, but you also become what your food eats.

How to Make Sure Your Animal Product are Truly "Free Range" and "Grass Fed"

Choosing organic animal products at the supermarket is miles better than eating the non-organic stuff. However, there is only one truly fail-safe way to make sure the meat and dairy products you and your family consume is truly organic and "free range" and "grass fed." You have to get to know your local farmer.

This is exactly what our great-grandparents did: they knew their local farmer and their local farmer knew them. That is truly a symbiotic food relationship! You would not want to purchase meat from a farmer who did not practice safe and healthy standards. Similarly, your local farmer does not want to harm his customers, since he not only has a relationship with his customers as individuals, but his possible carelessness could destroy his reputation and therefore his livelihood.

When you remove this intimate relationship between producer and consumer, the rules all change. When you have no access to the place where your food is grown or even no idea where your food comes from, there is no natural safety mechanism in place.

A farmer who lives and works a thousand miles away from you never sees where his product goes and honestly, today's CAFO-infested food supply, many probably don't care. This type of mercenary relationship only breeds greed, and puts the consumer at the bottom of the economic and safety chain.

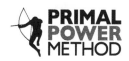

I know most of you are thinking that I am asking too much by insisting that you go see where your meat comes from, and become acquainted with the farmers who raise your food. Trust me; this is the best and perhaps only method to ensure that you are consuming a humanely raised and nutritionally dense meat or animal product.

Yet here is the best part: Once you establish this relationship, you are done. No more shopping from store to store trying to find the best cuts of meat from anonymous sources. When you create this type of "food relationship" you get the best food every single time, and you support your local economy—definitely a win/win outcome for everyone involved.

An Example of Sustainable Farming in Practice

Below is an excerpt from Joe Salatin's book *Folks, This Ain't Normal.* Salatin's description of the practices and policies implemented by his Polyface Farm is a good template to follow when searching for a reputable farmer following the practices to give you the best food products possible.

> In half a century, we've never bought a pound of chemical fertilizer and don't apply pesticides, herbicides, insecticides, or any other "-cide" to our plants and animals. Our animals don't do drugs. Instead we move them almost daily in a tightly choreographed ballet from pasture spot to pasture spot.

> They aren't confined in concentrated animal feeding operations. The herbivores receive no grain and the omnivores receive local, non-transgenic modified organism supplemental grains. We don't participate in any government programs, period. No cost share grants, no crop subsidies, no conservation easements, public or private. Our infrastructure is largely portable and nearly invisible.

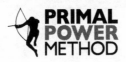

Nutritional Benefits of Going Organic

When it comes to quality there is just no comparison: organic is better. But beyond ethics, the real difference is in the nutritional value of organic "grass fed," "free range" animal products. Below are some simple facts regarding meat from these healthy sources.

- Compared with conventional beef, grass-fed is lower in saturated fat and higher in omega-3s, the heart-healthy fatty acids found in salmon. (Note that saturated fat is not "bad" – an important point I discuss at length in my previous book - but animals in nature simply tend to be leaner than their modern counterparts.)

- Pasture-fed cattle have lower levels of harmful Campylobacter and E. coli than those raised on CAFO farms.

- Calves raised on pasture have less harmful E. coli bacteria than calves raised in barns.

- Grass-finished cattle (cows that have eaten grass at the end of their pre-slaughter feeding process) excrete fewer dangerous bacteria in their feces; this reduces the spread of such bacteria onto meat in slaughterhouses.

- Grass-fed cattle get less sick less often and need fewer treatments with antibiotics.

Should this come as any surprise? Cows are meant to eat grass (not corn and soy!) and chickens are supposed to eat grass, seeds, and insects... not some contrived slurry of floor sweepings, engineered grains, bakery or distillery waste, and animal parts.

My Golden Rule for choosing meat? Remember that you are what you eat, and you also are *what your food has eaten!*

Pasture Raised Grass Fed Cows are Better for the Environment

Over the last decade the United Nations (UN) and environmental groups have declared war on the cow, implying that cattle are responsible for up

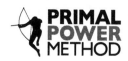

PRIMAL POWER METHOD

to 18 percent of all environmentally-unfriendly greenhouse gas emissions.

Do CAFO operations in the U.S. add to the greenhouse gasses and possibly global warming? At this time the answer is unclear, but is that really the point we should be focusing on?

It has been reported that a great deal of the greenhouse gas emissions attributed to cattle can really be attributed to the vast quantities of petrochemical inputs necessary to grow the grains used by CAFOs, the transportation of feed and cattle, and the release of gasses from enormous liquid manure lagoons on the modern factory farm.

In actuality when cows are raised as they are supposed to be (on open ranges eating indigenous grasses) this becomes a very different argument.

"Much of the carbon footprint of beef comes from growing grain to feed the animals, which requires fossil-fuel-based fertilizers, pesticides, transportation," writes Michael Pollan, author of *The Omnivore's Dilemma*. "Grass-fed beef has a much lighter carbon footprint."

Here's how traditionally-raised herds actually help support their immediate environment.

Remember, pastures are largely composed of perennial grasses—that is, plants that live for many years on the same rootstock.

When you rotate cattle and other ruminants (such as goats or sheep) across pastures full of these grasses, the grazing animals will cut the grass blades, which spurs new growth, while their trampling helps work manure and other decaying organic matter into the soil, turning it into rich humus. (Humus is decayed vegetable or animal matter that provides nutrients for plants.)

The plant's roots also help maintain soil health by retaining water and microbes. And healthy soil keeps carbon dioxide underground and out of the atmosphere.

It is estimated that 99 percent of U.S. beef cattle live out their last months on feedlots, where they are stuffed with corn and soybeans to add marbling of fat to their meat. Should we be surprised that this process causes harm to the environment?

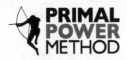

What is a Ruminant?

Ruminants are grazing animals that chew a cud (a portion of food that returns from a ruminant's stomach to the mouth to be chewed for the second time) and have split hooves. Ruminants include domestic cattle, bison, buffaloes, camels and llamas, giraffes, deer, pronghorns, antelopes, sheep, and goats.

These animals, except camels and llamas, have no upper front teeth; in place of teeth there is hardened gum, against which the lower front teeth bite. Ruminants hastily bite off and swallow their food (chiefly grasses, herbs, and twigs).

Grass Fed Cows Produce Better Milk

All of these principles apply to dairy products as well. For example, a study in the Journal of Dairy Science found:

Cows grazing pasture and receiving no supplemental feed had 500% more conjugated linoleic acid (CLA) in milk fat than cows fed typical dairy diets.

CLA has been found to:

- Increase metabolic rate
- Decrease abdominal fat
- Enhance muscle growth
- Lower cholesterol and triglycerides
- Lower insulin resistance
- Reduce food-induced allergic reactions
- Enhance your immune system

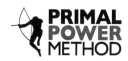

Note that not everyone can tolerate dairy products, and you certainly survive without them. However, if you digest them well and have access to organic options, I believe they can be a useful addition to a holistic, primal diet.

Better Products that are Better for You

For me the biggest difference when I switched to organic animal foods was a profound change in my digestion and digestive issues. When I consumed CAFO products I would undoubtedly have a couple mysterious stomach ailments a year and some of them were pretty bad, even requiring a doctor's visit. Once I made the change, I have not had even one of these bouts with organic meat and animal products. Let me repeat that, not one issue!

I eat my meat mostly medium/rare and it is delicious. I don't have to super char it to make sure I have killed the various organisms that can do me harm. People are amazed to find I let my meat sit out for hours getting to room temperature before I cook it. I cut my vegetables on the same plate after a simple water rinse, and can you believe it, I'm still alive! (Of course I do not necessarily recommend the above practice for you to follow; I have spent years improving my immune system in order to be able to prepare and consume my food in this manner.)

Once you make the change to organic "free range," "grass fed" products you will wonder why you ever purchased and consumed those CAFO products to begin with. Your health will improve, your stomach will feel better, and you will be helping the environment all in one swoop.

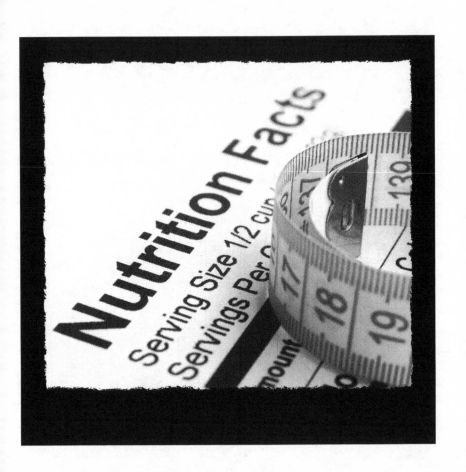

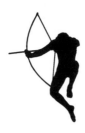

CHAPTER 6
THE SAVVY SHOPPER:
NAVIGATING FOOD LABELS

What an "Organic" Label Means

As previously mentioned, the USDA has created guidelines that food manufacturers must follow when labeling foods for sale in the U.S., so as to standardize the legal and practical term "organic." In this section, we will examine these regulations in detail. The good news is that once you understand what food labels really mean, it makes it so much easier to reach your nutrition and weight loss goals.

The following is the detailed version of how the USDA defines organic products, as taken directly from its website:

> Except for operations whose gross income from organic sales totals $5,000 or less, farm and processing operations that grow and process organic agricultural products must be certified by USDA-accredited certifying agents.
>
> Labeling requirements are based on the percentage of organic ingredients in a product.
>
> **Agricultural products labeled "100 percent organic" and "organic"**
>
> Products labeled as "100 percent organic" must contain (excluding water and salt) only organically produced ingredients and processing aids.
>
> Products labeled "organic" must consist of at least 95 percent organically produced ingredients (excluding water and salt). Any remaining product ingredients must consist of nonagricultural

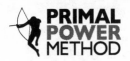

substances approved on the National List [*author's note: this is the list of "Allowed and Prohibited Substances" that identifies substances which may and may not be used in organic crop and livestock production*] including specific non-organically produced agricultural products that are not commercially available in organic form.

Products meeting the requirements for "100 percent organic" and "organic" may display these terms and the percentage of organic content on their principal display panel.

The USDA seal and the seal or mark of involved certifying agents may appear on product packages and in advertisements.

Agricultural products labeled "100 percent organic" and "organic" cannot be produced using excluded methods, sewage sludge, or ionizing radiation.

Processed products labeled "made with organic ingredients"

Processed products that contain at least 70 percent organic ingredients can use the phrase "made with organic ingredients" and list up to three of the organic ingredients or food groups on the principal display panel. For example, soup made with at least 70 percent organic ingredients and only organic vegetables may be labeled either "soup made with organic peas, potatoes, and carrots," or "soup made with organic vegetables."

Processed products labeled "made with organic ingredients" cannot be produced using excluded methods, sewage sludge, or ionizing radiation. The percentage of organic content and the certifying agent seal or mark may be used on the principal display panel. However, the USDA seal cannot be used anywhere on the package.

Processed products that contain less than 70 percent organic ingredients

These products cannot use the term organic anywhere on the principal display panel. However, they may identify the specific ingredients that are organically produced on the ingredients statement on the information panel.

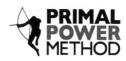

Other labeling provisions

Any product labeled as organic must identify each organically produced ingredient in the ingredient statement on the information panel.

The name of the certifying agent of the final product must be displayed on the information panel. The address of the certifying agent of the final product may be displayed on the information panel.

There are no restrictions on use of other truthful labeling claims such as "no drugs or growth hormones used," "free range," or "sustainably harvested."

So there you have it folks, that's what organic legally means in this country. Trust me, as someone who has read innumerable pages of Food and Drug Administration (FDA) and federal rules, policies and laws, this is about as straightforward as it gets. The government lawyers must have all been out playing golf the day this was drafted!

So here's a summary of what all that basically says. Products bearing the USDA Organic Seal simply signify the following:

1. It tells you that the grower/farmer has been inspected.

2. The inspector has verified that the producer of the food actually followed the Organic Standards, as outlined by the USDA.

3. The inspector works for a state or private agency accredited by the USDA.

4. All inspectors hold food producers to the same set of production standards as outlined in the USDA's National Organic Program.

Organic Certification from Agencies Other Than the USDA

Note that the USDA is not the only organization that may "certify" organic foods.

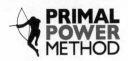

There are over 40 different organic certifiers worldwide, and many countries have their own certification standards and rules that they follow. This is not necessarily a bad thing, it's just something you need to be aware of so you can choose accordingly and wisely.

Because of the number of different types of certifications, and since we are based in the U.S., I have only covered the ones that apply in America. There is one other certification in the U.S. that I do feel is worth mentioning and you may come across at farmers' markets or small local grocery stores.

Certified Naturally Grown (CNG)

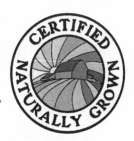

Certified Naturally Grown is a Grassroots Alternative to the USDA's National Organic Program meant primarily for small farmers distributing through local channels such as farmers' markets, roadside stands, local restaurants, community supported agriculture (CSA) programs, and small local grocery stores.

Certified Naturally Grown was created as a grassroots alternative to the USDA Organic program. It was created by small farmers, for small farmers.

Why? The USDA certification is often too much for many small farmers to afford, both in terms of money and paperwork requirements. This is even more true for farmers that grow a wide range of crops all at once, as is typical of a diversified family farm. This is one of the main reasons CNG was created: to give the small farmer an alternative to the USDA Certification.

To be granted the CNG certification, farmers must not use any synthetic herbicides, pesticides, fertilizers, antibiotics, hormones, or genetically modified organisms. CNG livestock are raised mostly on pasture and with space for freedom of movement. Feed must be grown without synthetic inputs or genetically modified seeds.

CNG is based on the participatory guarantee system (PGS) model in which inspections are typically carried out by other farmers. Carrying out an inspection is an annual work requirement of the CNG program. The PGS model promotes farmer-to-farmer knowledge sharing about best practices and fosters local networks that strengthen the farming community.

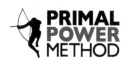

Another difference is that the Certified Naturally Grown certification process is transparent and open to the public--you will find every farmer's complete certification application online, as well as scanned copies of Inspection Summaries and Declarations.

Grass Fed, Free Range, and Organic: The Wise Choice

The food industry is not stupid; the moment they sense a trend rippling up through the marketplace they jump on it and dupe the consumer in the name of profit. They may simply slap the words "free range" or "grass fed" onto one of their product labels without changing much of anything about how they treat the animals except the sticker price for you.

And these days, there are a lot of products that have the words "grass fed," or "free range," or both, on their packages. However, without the "USDA Organic" or other legitimate organic label I consider these labels worthless.

Why? The words "grass fed" merely means the animals were fed grass. It does not tell you what kind of grass, whether the animals foraged for it themselves, if it was purchased feed grass (hay), if it was chemical-free, and so on.

Further, this designation does not guarantee that the animals were not given hormones or other drugs throughout their lives. So while I certainly want you to eat grass fed animals, the words on a label may themselves not be an assurance of excellent quality.

The same criticism can be made about the term "free range." This might conjure an image of cattle roaming a vast range in harmony with nature, but this label might merely mean that the animals had limited access to a cement paddock outdoors. Hardly ideal.

Moreover, the "free range" animals' diets could still have consisted of GMO feed, grains, or other highly processed, inappropriate food items that they were not meant to consume.

Food manufacturers usually couple these claims with the "natural" or "all-natural" label, which does demand some (legal) standards, but not enough for me to trust such products.

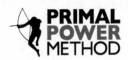

When it comes to the "USDA Certified Organic" label you know the producer had to follow a certain set of procedures in order get this certification on their meat product. You know there are no added hormones, no animal by-products in the feed rations, and all feed rations are organic products.

Now this is not to say the "organic" regulations are a perfect system. A cow fed organic grains (instead of grass) for most of its life is not a good thing; a grain-dominant ration is not a ruminant's natural diet, and vegetable feed could include corn and soy. So how do we alleviate this issue?

If I purchase any meat from a local store I make sure it is Certified USDA Organic, "grass fed," and "free range." Now without visiting your local farmer to check for yourself, there are some loopholes with these labels and that is just a fact of life. There is no way to tell for sure you are getting exactly what is claimed even on such a highly coveted organic label.

But it's certainly far better than the awful alternative: CAFO-raised animal products.

"All Natural?" Maybe, Maybe Not

I mentioned my apprehension at buying foods based on a label that claims the item is "natural." I'd like to explain why.

When it comes to causing the greatest amount of confusion among consumers trying to make healthy food choices, the term "all natural" is the winner.

As humans we tend to rely on this thing we call "trust," so when we see a food item labeled as "all natural," we expect it to be… all natural.

Unfortunately the food industry and its billions of dollars of influence on the federal government have shamelessly betrayed the consumer's trust in this regard, turning the "all natural" label into an utter travesty… and, I hope, reinforcing the much more realistic motto of "*caveat emptor*" or "buyer beware" in its place.

I also fell for the false assurance of the "all natural" label conferred on food products and assumed these foods were superior, safe products.

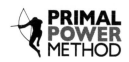

My tenure at the FDA opened my eyes to just what "all natural" really means (or in this case, doesn't mean!).

You see, most people confuse "all natural" with "organic," which couldn't be further from the truth.

Would you be surprised to learn that there is *no actual official or legal definition* of what the "all natural" designation means in the food industry? In other words, it pretty much means nothing.

Basically if you see "all natural" or "natural" on any food item (other than meat or poultry, which we will discuss next) it means absolutely nothing. The product does not necessarily contain ingredients of superior quality, and is not regulated any differently than a food that does not have these magical descriptions on their label.

I find it interesting that this claim would even have to be made on a food label, since it stands to reason that all of our food should be "all natural." Yet in today's food industry real food is getting harder and harder to find. The plights of our health and our food are directly related: the more garbage they put out as food, the more of it we eat, the fatter and sicker we get, and all the while the industry gets richer.

What a deal!

The Meat and Poultry Exception

There is one area where the term "natural" is regulated. Only meat and poultry products have any USDA rules that apply when using the terms "natural" or "all natural." These rules are:

1. The meat must have no artificial flavors, colors, chemical preservatives, or other synthetic ingredients.

2. The meat must be only minimally processed. ("Minimal processing" means that the product was processed in a manner that does not fundamentally alter the product.)

3. The companies have to define what is meant by the term(s) "natural" or "all natural" on their package labels, such as including the words "no antibiotics or no hormones."

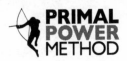

For years the food industry has used these confusing terms and sleight of hand to charge more for products labeled in this manner and has duped many a consumer into believing these were superior products.

Of course, the term "natural" may just as easily be on a quality product. Why? There are also honest companies that simply cannot afford to secure an official USDA Certification for their products and they will use the "all natural" or "made with all natural ingredients" designation on their label instead.

This is when you have to do your research and decide if the company making such a claim is actually following through on what their labels promise.

You Scratch my Back...

The unit that deals with meat and poultry in the USDA is the Food Safety and Inspection Service (FSIS). Would you be surprised to learn that FSIS has a long history of "a gentlemen's agreement" with the large meat industry lobby groups? Yeah, me neither.

Naturally Raised

Hot on the heels of the "all natural" bandwagon is the phrase "naturally raised."

The term "naturally raised" is a voluntary marketing claim that manufacturers can choose to use on labels of meat and meat products.

Legally, it means that livestock have been raised entirely without growth promotants, which are supplements of naturally occurring hormones used by some producers to increase weight gain and improve feed efficiency in cattle. They have also been raised without antibiotics (except for reasons of parasite control), and have never been fed animal or aquatic byproducts derived from slaughter or harvest processes.

If a manufacturer chooses to use this term, it must be able to provide evidence to support the claim. Note that the term has *no relevance to animal welfare.*

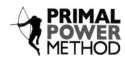

Other Common Terms on Food Labels

Beyond the terms "organic" and "natural," there are a plethora of other marketing claims on food packaging. Here's what the most common ones really mean.

Certified: The term "certified" implies that the USDA's Food Safety and Inspection Service and the Agriculture Marketing Service have officially evaluated a meat product for class, grade, or other quality characteristics (e.g., "Certified Angus Beef"). When used under other circumstances, the term must be closely associated with the name of the organization responsible for the "certification" process, e.g., "XYZ Company's Certified Beef."

No Hormones (pork or poultry): Hormones are not allowed in raising hogs or poultry. Therefore, the claim "no hormones added" is true for all pork and poultry sold in the U.S.! To mitigate this redundancy, the term cannot be used to describe pork or poultry products unless it is followed by a statement that says "federal regulations prohibit the use of hormones."

No Hormones (beef): The term "no hormones administered" may be approved for use on the label of beef products, if sufficient documentation is provided to the USDA by the producer showing that no hormones have been used in raising the animals.

No Antibiotics (red meat and poultry): The terms "no antibiotics added" may be used on labels for meat or poultry products, if sufficient documentation is provided by the producer to the USDA demonstrating that the animals were raised without antibiotics.

Free Range or Free Roaming: Producers must demonstrate to the USDA that the poultry has been allowed access to the outside.

This can be misleading, as it just means that the animals have access to go outside. It doesn't necessarily mean they ever made it outside, and "outside" could simply be an outdoor slab of concrete.

Pasture Raised: This term, sometimes referred to as "access to pasture," is regulated as part of the National Organic Program of the USDA.

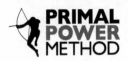

Manufacturers who use this label must meet certain requirements, such as providing year-round access to the outdoors for all ruminant animals, providing them with pasture throughout the grazing season in their area and ensuring that the animals get at least 30 percent of their dry-feed intake from pasture grazing over the course of grazing season.

Cage Free: Under USDA regulations, this means that laying hens live un-caged, typically within a barn, warehouse, building, or other enclosed area. They must have unlimited access to food and water and the freedom to roam within the enclosed area during their egg-production cycle. Note that *cage-free does **not** mean the hens have access to the outdoors*. Cage-free birds can engage in some natural behaviors, such as nesting and spreading their wings. However, practices such as beak cutting are allowed.

Poultry raised for their meat are rarely caged; this term usually applies more to laying (egg-producing) hens.

Grass Fed: Grass and forage shall be the feed source consumed for the lifetime of the ruminant animal, with the exception of milk consumed prior to weaning. The diet shall be derived solely from forage consisting of grass (annual and perennial), forbs (e.g., legumes, Brassica), browse, or cereal grain crops in the vegetative (pre-grain) state.

Animals cannot be fed grain or grain byproducts and must have continuous access to pasture during the growing season. Hay, haylage, baleage, silage, crop residue without grain, and other roughage sources may also be included as acceptable feed sources. Routine mineral and vitamin supplementation may also be included in the feeding regimen.

If incidental supplementation occurs due to inadvertent exposure to non-forage feedstuffs or to ensure the animal's well being at all times during adverse environmental or physical conditions, the producer must fully document (e.g., receipts, ingredients, and tear tags) the supplementation that occurs including the amount, the frequency, and the supplements provided.

Grain Fed: Under the United States Grain Standards Act (GSA; 57 FR 3274; January 29, 1992) and therefore acceptable to be included in the diet as grain are barley, canola, corn, flaxseed, mixed grain, oats, rye, sorghum, soybeans, sunflower seed, triticale, and wheat, and any other food grains, feed grains, and oilseeds for which standards are established under section 76 of the GSA.

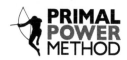

Additional feedstuffs that are acceptable to be included in the diet as grain for AMS administered USDA Certified or USDA Audit and Accreditation Programs are rice, millet, amaranth, buckwheat, and distiller's grain (with or without solubles).

Note: You should avoid consuming meat from ruminant animals that have been fed strictly or mainly a grain diet as it makes them sick. They are given large doses of antibiotics in order to counteract this type of diet. In addition, grain fed usually means a diet high in corn and soy that we know is mainly GMO produced in the U.S. Choose organic and grass fed!

Certified Humane: This is a voluntary certification and labeling program administered by Humane Farm Animal Care to ensure humane treatment of farm animals from birth through slaughter. Other organizations also offer certification and labeling programs. This term is not regulated by the USDA.

Certified producers must meet species standards for such things as space, shelter, handling, fresh water, and a diet free of added hormones and antibiotics. Cages, crates and tie stalls are prohibited.

Animals must be able to engage in natural behaviors. For instance, chickens must be able to spread their wings and dust bathe, while pigs must have space to move around and root.

Vegetarian Fed: This term isn't regulated by the USDA. It is generally meant to suggest that an animal is fed a healthier diet and is raised without being fed animal byproducts or dairy products. According to the USDA, manufacturers that use this term on package labels must be able to provide evidence to support the claim.

This has become a popular label, especially on chicken egg boxes. Here is my opinion on this matter.

This type of label probably came about just as the grain fed label did. There has been growing public concern about meat, most especially during the "mad cow" scare when it became more widely known that big industry cattle farms were feeding cows slaughterhouse cattle remains. So in order to put the consumer at ease the "grain fed" label was created.

At around the same time the equally gruesome fact that factory farm chickens were being fed chicken remains was revealed. So it seems

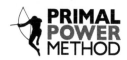
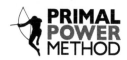

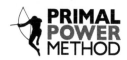

91

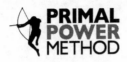

logical that food manufacturers would put this label on chicken products so as to alleviate the concerns of consumers.

However, there is a problem with the vegetarian designation for chickens since chickens are not naturally vegetarians but omnivores, meaning they also consume protein from non-plant sources, usually in the form of insects and worms.

So if you want to consume the best eggs they must come from free-range, organic raised chickens. Be aware that just as in the example of grain-fed cows, "vegetarian-fed chickens" usually means the birds' feed is high in soy and corn, and is almost certainly GMO, since it is the cheapest type of feed.

Many consumers have been duped by the "vegetarian fed" label; I know I was until I discovered what it meant. One company made the mistake of actually putting what the vegetarian feed consisted of on the back of one of their packages of chicken thighs that I bought. Sure enough, soy and corn were right there on the label.

This is especially troubling when you are trying to avoid GMO and soy products, due to health concerns or food allergies. Remember that what your food eats is what you end up eating as well. If they are eating soy, so are you.

You Are What Your Food Eats

Are you confused yet? Well, that is exactly what these labels are intended to do—keep you in the dark about what is actually in your food.

To drive the importance of organic animal products home, I think it is easier to take a look at what is actually allowed in the feed of conventional animal products (see below). This is why I preach going organic; it makes your food choices a whole lot simpler, and you only have to look for one label.

Dairy cows – antibiotics, pig and chicken byproducts, hormones (for growth), pesticides, sewage sludge.

Beef cows – antibiotics, pig and chicken byproducts, steroids, hormones, pesticides, sewage sludge.

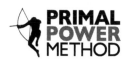

Pigs – antibiotics, animal byproducts, pesticides, sewage sludge, arsenic-based drugs (growth hormones are prohibited).

Broiler chickens – antibiotics, animal byproducts, pesticides, sewage sludge, arsenic-based drugs (growth hormones are prohibited).

Egg laying hens – antibiotics, animal byproducts, pesticides, sewage sludge, arsenic-based drugs.

Remember, you are what you eat, and you become what your food eats. Enough said.

A Note About Labels on Produce

Now that you know about animal products in depth, there is one more detail about labels on fruits and vegetables that I want you to have in your toolkit.

There is an easy way to determine if a plant-based item is GMO or organic. Look at the PLU code – that's the little sticker found on fruits and vegetables.

If a fruit or vegetable has only 4 digits in its PLU code, it is conventionally grown and may be genetically engineered. If it has 5 numbers and starts with an 8, then it is GMO. However, if it starts with a 9, it is organic.

When shopping for fruits and vegetables I always search for that little sticker and make sure it starts with a 9. I have purchased fruits and vegetables in the organic section only to notice once I arrived home that they were not organic because the sticker PLU code did not start with a 9. You must be ever vigilant, as non-organic products will almost always be displayed right next to their non-organic counterparts.

Also note that, unfortunately, the "8" notation for GMO produce is only voluntary, as is the use of all PLU codes. Consequently many (if not all) purveyors of food items don't bother to reveal GMO-related information to consumers.

Here's the bottom line on food labels: they don't usually mean what they would seem to imply. Instead of trying to figure it all out, just look for the "organic" food label and you'll be doing yourself (and probably some helpless animals) a huge service!

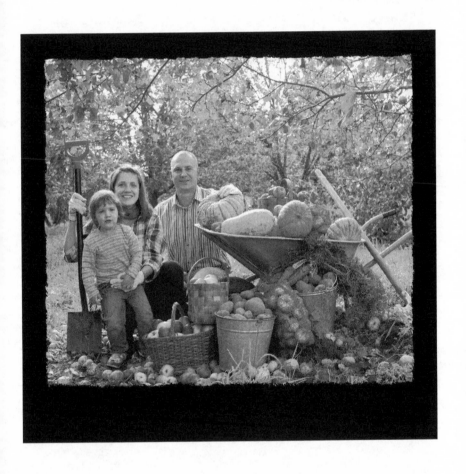

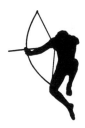

CHAPTER 7
SIMPLE WAYS TO START YOUR ORGANIC JOURNEY

So by now I hope that you have been inspired to start introducing organic foods in your diet. Let's talk about the best way to go about making the change.

Most people think they must jump into the organic world headfirst and buy all organically-made products right away.

This sounds great, but in reality it is very difficult to do. It takes time to learn where, how, and from whom to by organic products. Unfortunately there is no one-stop-shop for buying organic products and foods; it takes time to locate all of your favorite products. It can be overwhelming and discouraging if done all at once.

The Primal Power Approach

This kind of dilemma is why I developed the five principles of the Primal Power Method, as outlined in the introduction to this book (and discussed in detail in my previous book):

1. Knowledge is power
2. Avoid extremes
3. Keep it simple
4. Something is better than nothing
5. Take action today and every day

These emphasize that the Method is all about the real rather than simply the ideal. In this spirit I encourage you to avoid an extreme approach to going organic. Let's think about how you can make the change slowly but surely, in small and realistic steps.

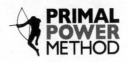

There is an easy way to get started, and that is with the so-called "dirtiest" and "cleanest" produce choices. You can lower your pesticide intake substantially by avoiding the non-organic versions of the most pesticide-contaminated fruits and vegetables and eating the least contaminated non-organic produce instead.

In other words, by purchasing fruits and vegetables that may not be organic, but are typically much lower in pesticide residues (i.e. are "cleaner") and by avoiding the ones that are considered to be the most toxic (i.e. the "dirtiest"), and choosing their organic versions in their place, you'll already be ahead of the game.

This way as you are learning and finding your way you can get these "lesser offenders" at your everyday grocery store and embark on the path to become more comfortable with organic shopping habits.

Below is the list of the best and worst fruits and vegetables in regards to pesticide exposure, by the Environmental Working Group, current as of this writing (2012; the list is updated annually on the group's website, www.ewg.org.)

Dirtiest (Most pesticides – buy organic)

1. Apples
2. Celery
3. Sweet bell peppers
4. Peaches
5. Strawberries
6. Nectarines (imported)
7. Grapes
8. Spinach
9. Lettuce
10. Cucumbers
11. Blueberries (domestic)
12. Potatoes
13. Green beans
14. Kale

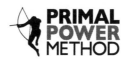

Cleanest (Lowest in pesticides – okay to choose non-organic for now)

1. Onions
2. Sweet corn
3. Pineapple
4. Avocado
5. Cabbage
6. Sweet peas
7. Asparagus
8. Mangoes
9. Egg plant
10. Kiwi
11. Cantaloupe
12. Sweet potatoes
13. Grapefruit
14. Watermelon
15. Mushrooms

Of course your goal should be to incorporate as many organic foods and produce into your life as possible. But I have found the above list to be helpful for people just getting started on the road to health and wellness and for those times when we don't have access to organic foods, such as when traveling.

A note of caution: remember that just because the "clean" foods on this list may be low in pesticides, it doesn't mean they are not GMO products. And of course they are likely to have been grown with synthetic fertilizers. Refer back to the GMO chapter of this book for a list of common GMO products.

Also, try to avoid all non-organic corn as the majority of it grown in the U.S. is genetically modified.

But Isn't it Expensive to Eat Healthy?

Many of you may say that this all sounds great in a perfect world, but you just can't afford to eat healthfully as it would be too expensive.

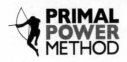

Happily, as some of you may have learned from the groundbreaking Primal Power Method series, this excuse simply doesn't hold water when you get down to the facts.

I'm sure most of you have seen reports, articles, or documentaries devised to make you feel sorry for poor, sick people who just can't afford healthy food.

These programs and articles always portray a poor family who just can't afford organic fruits, vegetables, and meat for their family, so they have to eat fast food as the only way they can survive economically. These families are typically shown going to some local fast food chain and ordering off the dollar menu. The total bill for a family of four ends up being between $20-$25 dollars.

However, that doesn't sound like such a good deal to me, especially when you know they have been limited to the cheapest items—both in price and nutritional punch—on the menu.

Compare this strategy to preparing a healthy organic meal from whole, fresh ingredients at home, and the truly better deal from all angles becomes immediately apparent. For example, I can purchase 10-12 organic free-range chicken legs, organic salad greens, and some organic fruit for $10-$15 dollars total. And I can prepare all of this in less time than it takes you to get in your car go through the drive through and return home. Not only did I save you money on your meal, you didn't have to spend money on gas either!

Unfortunately the poor family depicted in these examples as well as others like them all around our country are not only malnourished, but are nearly always obese.

And we wonder why we have a health epidemic in America today. One thing is certain; if you constantly bombard your body with chemicals and mass-produced food you will suffer… and suffer mightily.

There are many other great ways to save money on a budget, yet still incorporate a few or, preferably, many organic food selections on a budget. A quick web search will reveal many ideas, and all of them apply to organic foods as well. For example, you can clip coupons for organic foods just as easily as you can for non-organic foods.

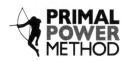

There's a lot of great eating-on-a-budget advice out there. Here are a few other highlights to get you started:

For organic produce:

- Instead of purchasing based on recipes, plan your recipes around what's on sale and cheapest that week. Typically, this will be food that is in-season. Scan the weekly flyers from your local grocery store to help plan meals around the organic food sales before you buy.

- Get good at preparing the vegetables that are cheapest in your region. In many parts of America, these include onions, carrots, potatoes, cabbages, squash, beets... you know, the stuff most of our grandparents cooked!

- Buy frozen organic vegetables when they are on sale and save them for some quick meal fixes. Fresh food is better but frozen works well in a pinch without sacrificing too much nutrition.

- Some grocery stores have a day of the week that fresh produce items that are about to expire are heavily discounted. Similarly, some vendors at farmer's markets will cut prices in the last half hour of the market in order to get rid of product that would otherwise just go to waste. Ask around to see when these times are and take advantage of them. Incidentally, this typically also applies to meats and dairy items in grocery stores.

For organic animal products:

- Buy organic meat from your local farmer in bulk, and freeze it. Many small organic farmers are happy to sell their product in very large portions at a steep discount.

- Ask your local farmer if they process their animals on site, and if they offer a discount to those able to come pick it up as they harvest. This especially applies to poultry farmers, who are able to rent mobile processing vans that come to their farms. On processing day, the farmers are often willing to sell the birds at a discount on site, after processing but before freezing.

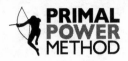

- Get skilled at preparing the cheapest cuts of meat. These are usually the organ meats (such as liver) and tough cuts of meat like the shoulder blade of the animal. Learn how to slow cook these in an oven or, even more easily, in a crock pot. Done right, these are just a delicious as filet mignon but at a fraction of the price, and really not that much more difficult to prepare.

For more simple, money- and time-saving menu ideas, check out my companion book: *Primal Power Method: Quick, Super-Easy Primal and Paleo Meal Recipes*. It makes preparing inexpensive, whole food meals simple and achievable for even the most inexperienced of home cooks.

Why Organic May Not Be Enough

Of course if your current diet consists of mostly poor food choices, it won't be enough to merely substituting organic products for all the same convenience foods you have always eaten. As outlined in my other books and blog, you still have to make wise choices.

An organic cookie, after all, is still a cookie!

But is an organic cookie better for you than one made with highly processed chemicals and ingredients? It is, but it also contains large amounts of all the things you should be avoiding to attain optimal health.

These are mainly sugar and high amounts of refined carbohydrates, which are greatly responsible for our current health and obesity epidemic (I discuss why in depth in my other writings.)

I have lost count of the people I have met over the years who eat an organic diet and just can't figure out why they are overweight and don't feel as well as they should.

Well, when I peel back the layers of their supposedly healthy way of eating I always find plenty of the same foods that are making everyone sick: processed carbohydrates and sugar.

That's partly why I wrote this book: Buying and living an organic lifestyle is more than just throwing something that says "organic" or "all natural" into your shopping cart. It always comes down to making the right food choices.

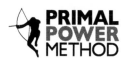

Here's another example of well-meaning but misguided intentions. How many of you have purchased gluten-free items in order to lose weight? I know I have met many people who actually think gluten-free eating is a weight-loss diet.

A gluten-free diet is in fact a means to avoid a component of wheat, or other grains, which in some people triggers allergic or autoimmune responses to foods that contain gluten.

But through aggressive marketing, misleading media and food company hype surrounding gluten-free products, people have wasted a great deal of time and money believing they can have the body of a model by following yet another misguided trend.

Don't get me wrong, going gluten free is critical for most, but most of today's gluten-free products are carb or sugar bombs in disguise. Also most gluten-free products found in your grocery store are not truly gluten-free. They are "technically" gluten-free because they do not contain the molecule gluten, but they do contain a very close relative of gluten causing the same problems as gluten. Choose wisely.

Putting It All Together

I think by now you can agree that trying to pursue an organic eating plan can be confusing if you don't have the right information. Food companies have bombarded us with slogans and labeling practices to keep us guessing as to what's really in their products. But now that you are armed with the facts you know what all that misleading information really means on those labels.

What will you actually do with this valuable information?

Probably the most important part of "going organic" is figuring out where to find truly organic food items. Take it from me, you will not be able to figure it all out over night, instead you will have to find a system that works for you.

Unfortunately there is no really good one-stop-shop when it comes to organic food, and you will have to piece it together, but I hope the information I give you below will make the process simpler.

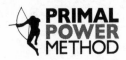

Local Grocery Stores and Markets that Support an Organic and Healthy Lifestyle

With the popularity of natural and organic products, more and more grocery chains have popped up over the last decade supporting this type of lifestyle.

If possible I recommend you get the bulk of your healthy and organic foods from your local farmers for the various reasons we have already covered. But for those of you living in a more metropolitan or non-farm-friendly area this just may not be possible. In addition, there are numerous local health-oriented grocery stores nationwide that will usually carry far more locally grown items, labeled as such.

Below I have provided you with a list below of what I feel are the best food store chains carrying products that support a healthier lifestyle.

Trader Joe's

Trader Joe's is a national chain (currently in nine states). It carries some conventional foods as well as natural and organic food. The company is known for carrying unusual products, and many of the items they sell are the Trader Joe's brand. The company tries to source items locally, so not all products are available in all locations.

Whole Foods

Whole Foods Market has over 300 stores in the United States and United Kingdom combined. Headquartered in Austin, Texas this large chain is available in most of the states in the United States.

Sprouts

Sprouts, like Trader Joe's, carries both organic and conventional foods with a focus on fresh, local items. With over 150 locations, the store carries bulk items, natural cosmetics, and a variety of meats as well as produce, canned, and frozen goods.

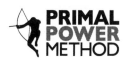

A common mistake people make when converting to organic and natural products is they go to these grocery chains and do not change their shopping habits. So instead of making healthier food choices, which is what will ultimately change one's health for the better, they take the easy route. But buying organic processed pizzas and cookies will not make you healthier in the end!

Taking it a Step Further:
The Benefits of "Eating Local"

We have previously touched on the idea of getting to know your local farmers. Well, once you have started including more organic foods from grocery stores into your meals, I would encourage you to experiment with purchasing locally-grown foods from your area.

Keep in mind that, when only a small number of factory farms control and centralize our meat, or American agriculture as a whole for that matter, your food has to travel long distances to reach you.

Back when small local farmers ruled the land, your food just had to travel from the farm to your local market, usually in your immediate vicinity. Now food is commonly transported great distances to get to your table. This is one of the main reasons these mass farming operations must continually cut costs on raising the animals: because they also have to deal with transportation costs that didn't exist a century ago.

It is estimated that over 13 percent of total global warming is attributed to the transportation of food. Our favorite mega-"farm", the CAFO, uses large amounts of energy transporting feed rations and transporting animals to feedlots and to slaughter. Then, the meat must be shipped to centralized distribution centers, and finally to the stores for consumers to purchase.

The U.S. is one of the worst offenders in this regard. In 2011, the U.S. exported and imported over 2 billion pounds of beef and veal according to the United States Department of Agriculture.

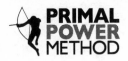

I don't know about you, but this makes no sense to me! We are exporting and importing almost the same amount of beef and veal; yes, this is insanity! I'm sure this is through some great export/import legislation concocted by our increasingly unpopular Congress. We are burning billions of gallons of fuel, and wasting every type of energy source we have worldwide, for a no net change in our meat supplies?

These billions of pounds of meat being shipped around the world are not only wasting valuable energy, (which you and I pay for in higher energy and food prices in the end) but they also drastically add to our carbon footprint.

The same principle applies to product. Have you noticed your grocery tomatoes coming from places such as Chile, Argentina and other locations half way across the world? I live in Southern California and I'm pretty sure we can grow tomatoes almost all year around, yet many local chain stores have them from every imaginable destination except for California, or even the U.S., for that matter.

It's complete and utter insanity!

Fortunately there is a growing trend of small, traditional polyculture-based farming taking place in this country. In some places these farms are obvious, and in others you may need to drive a few miles to find them. But they are out there and they need our support!

Let's stop sending our food on international itineraries before we eat it! Here are ten great reasons to buy your food locally:

1. Locally grown food tastes better. Food grown in your own community is usually picked within the past day or two. It's crisp, sweet, and loaded with flavor. Produce flown or trucked in is much older. Several studies have shown that the average distance food travels from farm to plate is 1,500 miles.

2. Local produce is better for you. Fresh produce loses nutrients quickly. Locally grown food, purchased soon after harvest, retains its nutrients.

3. Local food preserves genetic diversity. In the modern industrial agricultural system, varieties are chosen for their ability to ripen

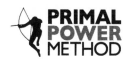

simultaneously and withstand harvesting equipment. Only a handful of varieties of fruits and vegetables meet those rigorous demands, so there is little genetic diversity in the plants grown. Local farms, in contrast, grow a huge number of varieties to provide a long season of harvest, an array of eye-catching colors, and the best flavors.

4. Local food is virtually always GMO-free. Although biotechnology companies have been trying to commercialize genetically modified fruits and vegetables, they are currently licensing them only to large factory-style farms. Local farmers don't have access to genetically modified seed, and most of them wouldn't use it even if they could.

5. Local food supports local farm families (your neighbors). With fewer than one million Americans now listing farming as their primary occupation, farmers are a vanishing breed. Local farmers who sell direct to consumers cut out the middle man and get full retail price for their crops.

6. Local food builds a stronger community. When you buy direct from the farmer, you are re-establishing a time-honored connection between the eater and the grower.

7. Local food preserves open space. As the value of direct-marketed fruits and vegetables increases, selling farmland for development becomes less likely. The rural landscape will survive only as long as farms are financially viable.

8. Local food helps to keep your taxes in check. Farms contribute more in taxes than they require in services, whereas suburban development costs more than it generates in taxes.

9. Local food supports a clean environment and benefits wildlife. A well-managed family farm is a place where the resources of fertile soil and clean water are valued. Good stewards of the land grow cover crops to prevent erosion and replace nutrients used by their crops. Cover crops also capture carbon emissions and help combat global warming.

10. Local food is about the future. By supporting local farmers today, you can help ensure that there will be farms in your community tomorrow, so that future generations will have access to nourishing, flavorful, and abundant food.

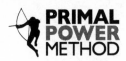

Community Supported Agriculture (CSAs)

Now that we know most of our food travels thousands of miles to market, is doused with chemical fertilizers, herbicides and pesticides, and grown in substandard soils, what can we do about it?

The easiest way for you to support you local farming economy and get well-priced, healthy food is by belonging to a community supported agriculture (CSA) association or group. CSAs have been around for a long time, but most people have never heard of them or even know what they are.

What is a CSA and How Does it Work?

Community supported agriculture is basically a local farmer, or group of farmers, who offer a certain number of "shares" to the public. Typically the share consists of a box or container of vegetables made available weekly, but on some occasions other farm products may be included.

Consumers can purchase a share, membership, or subscription. It just depends on how the farmer has their system set up. Farmers who specialize in raising animals also sell shares, in which you will receive meat and dairy products from that farmer.

Most CSAs operate in the following manner: You first must apply to belong to a particular CSA, and since they have a limited number of members they can support you may have to be put on a waiting list. Once you become a member you pay for your share quarterly and will regularly receive a small or large box of various fruits and vegetables.

You may receive your box once a week, or every two weeks, or sometimes once a month depending on your needs. I recommend people start with the small box every two weeks until you can figure out how much you or your family will need. Also as you incorporate a healthier lifestyle you will probably start to increase the size of the box or the frequency of your pick-ups.

One main point people need to understand about CSAs, especially when it comes to fruits and vegetables, is that these are not grocery stores. You will not be able to choose what you want; what you get is what you get. This means you will be receiving fruits and vegetables that are in

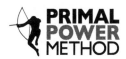

season and subject to whatever weather and other natural events that the season brings. In other words, you will not be able to get strawberries in December or asparagus in August.

Some CSA's are more flexible and will give you some options, but most operate by the premise of everyone gets the same items at every pick-up. The good news is that the internet offers many ideas and tips about how to prepare different types of produce, so if you are not familiar with every vegetable that arrives in your CSA share you can easily learn how to use it. Or, check out some of the vegetable ideas in my Primal Power Method meal guide, available from the Primal Power Method website. You can mix and match lots of different vegetables into the recipe ideas I outline in the guide.

Meat and dairy CSAs are usually more flexible and allow you to select different meat items. For instance the CSA I belong to in San Diego, California (www.da-le-ranch.com) has gotten to know me over the years and my meat share is pretty much tailored to my preferences.

For people looking to incorporate more organic foods into their lifestyle I highly recommend joining a CSA. First you will be surprised at the amount of food you will receive for the price; it is often much cheaper than shopping at your local grocery store. Secondly you will be forced to experiment and eat foods you have never eaten before; I know this is the case with me. Finally it removes much of the confusion and time commitment devoted to grocery shopping, since you just turn up to get your box of goodies at a designated pick-up point—it's that simple.

A Word of Caution

Not all CSAs are created equal, and not every CSA program will follow the practices you may prefer. For example, some CSAs still use chemical fertilizers, pesticides, and herbicides.

Any CSA worth its salt will tell you on their website or application how they grow and raise their products. Luckily for me the CSA closest to my house also provides a majority of the USDA Certified Organic fruits and vegetables in my area.

This being said a great number of CSA's that adhere to sustainable, organic farming principles are not "USDA Certified Organic" as it is just

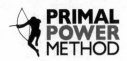

too expensive for smaller farming operations to obtain the certification. This is where your due diligence comes into play; most will allow you to tour the farm and see how they operate. Try doing that at a Tyson or Cargill farm!

A good example is that is that very few meat and dairy CSAs are USDA Certified Organic. The costs are astronomical for small animal farms to get this certification. The CSA I belong to where I get my meat products is not USDA Certified Organic, but I know they use the practices I'm looking for in a meat producing farm and that is good enough for me. When you go to a farm it's pretty obvious if the animals are being well cared for or not!

That is probably the biggest difference between belonging to a CSA and purchasing your food items from a local grocery store: a one-on-one, personal relationship with the farmer and the food you eat.

How to Find a CSA

To find a CSA in your area, try an internet search or via various data base websites that have CSAs listed in a certain area or all over the country. The best one I have found and used over the years is www.LocalHarvest. org. Local Harvest has a searchable database of farmers' markets, family farms and other sources of sustainably grown food, which offer organic produce, grass-fed meats and other foods.

In addition, please see our list of various organizations specializing in finding organic and natural foods in the Appendix of this book.

What to look for in a CSA

Make sure the CSA you opt to support offers foods that meet the following criteria:

1. Grown without pesticides and chemical fertilizers (organic foods fit this description, but so do some non-organic foods).

2. Not genetically modified (GMO).

3. Contains no added growth hormones, antibiotics, or other drugs.

4. Does not contain artificial anything, nor any preservatives.

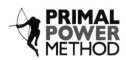

5. Fresh (if you have to choose between wilted organic produce or fresh conventional produce, the latter may be the better option).

6. Did not come from a factory farm.

7. Grown with the laws of nature in mind (meaning animals are fed their native diets, not a mix of grains and animal byproducts, and have free-range access to the outdoors).

8. Grown in a sustainable way (using minimal amounts of water, protecting the soil from burnout, and turning animal wastes into natural fertilizers instead of environmental pollutants).

Farmers' Markets

Another great way to find local organic and healthy foods is to visit and shop at a farmers' market.

In the last decade the local farmers' market has become increasingly popular and the favorite marketing venue for many farmers throughout the United States, as well as a pleasant weekly ritual for many shoppers. Farmers' markets are considered one of the oldest forms of direct marketing by small local farmers.

Farmers' markets tend to have a lot more items than just fruits, vegetables, meat, and dairy products. You will see items ranging from flowers to clothing items and jewelry, as well as great local food.

In a farmers' market, a group of farmers sell their products once or twice a week at a designated public place like a park or parking lot. Some farmers' markets have live entertainment. Shopping at a farmers' market is a great way to meet local farmers, your neighbors, and find fresh, flavorful produce.

CSAs and farmers' markets are no different from any other source of your family's food: you have to do your due diligence. Just because someone has a booth at a farmers' market does not mean they are following the ecological and health practices you are looking for in your food items. Interview them and find out what you need to know. Many farmers who have CSAs also participate in your local farmers' markets as well.

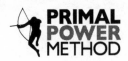

The great benefit of local farmers' markets is they offer a great deal of diversity in organic and natural products. For example, they are a great place to find local raw honey, which is preferred by most holistic health care practitioners because allergies or reactions can occur from other honey due to unfamiliar pollen from distant locations.

How to Get Started at a Farmer's Market

I do not recommend people just starting out on the path to an organic lifestyle to jump right into a farmers' market. The reason for caution here is that you need to be a little more experienced to be able to pick out the good items from the not-so-good items.

Farmers' markets can be overwhelming for the beginner, but I do not want to discourage organic-food-novices. For the first couple visits, just walk around and become familiar with the sellers and various booths and products.

As with CSAs, the best place to search for farmer's markets is through www.LocalHarvest.org. Local Harvest has a searchable database of farmers' markets, family farms, and other sources of sustainably grown food, which offer produce, grass-fed meats, and other foods.

A Summary of Steps Towards an Organic Lifestyle

1. Remember that transitioning from the typical Western Diet of highly processed foods to natural and organic foods takes time. Don't try to make all the changes all at once. By incorporating them slowly you will be able to avoid food allergies and intolerances.

2. The best place to start is at a local supermarket with an organics section and replacing some of your fruits and vegetables with USDA Certified Organic choices (especially choosing substitutes for those listed on the EWG's list of dirtiest fruits and vegetables).

3. Once you become comfortable selecting organic fruits and vegetables at your local grocery store chain start looking for a CSA you can join. Again stick with just fruits and vegetables, learn how to prepare them, and incorporate the new items into your daily menu.

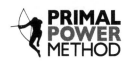

4. For hard-to-find items, or items your CSA does not carry, shop at local health food markets and grocery stores.

5. Incorporate the larger retail organic-carrying markets if needed and use them when on the road or if your work requires you to travel a great deal.

6. Experiment with some of the all-natural and organic meats and dairy products at your local stores. Remember they are far more expensive in stores, but this is to get you comfortable with choosing the healthier versions of these products.

7. Once you have become comfortable purchasing organic fruits and vegetables, start looking for local meat and dairy farmers. These are usually more difficult to find than fruit and vegetable CSAs and is why I recommend saving this for later. In addition, the vendors or CSA you belong to will be able to steer you in the right direction and will probably save you a lot of time.

Another Option: Making an Organic Garden at Home

Many people today are interested in raising some of the food they eat right in their own yards at home. This trend is probably inspired by many impulses, including the wish to avoid contaminated produce from distant, unknown sources, the wish to save money on food, and the simple pleasure of picking and eating delicious ripe fruit and vegetables from just outside one's door.

An organic garden at home can also be a most pleasant means to teach children about biology and ecology and at the same time instill in them a love of tending the earth, an appreciation for the genuine flavors of fruits and vegetables in their natural state of readiness, and the invigorating spirit of independence and self-reliance.

Creating your own organic home garden is easier than you may think, and doesn't necessarily require a great deal of space. Your garden will do best if the spot you choose receives full sun for at least eight hours a day—and certain plants, such as sweet corn and melons, will prefer even more.

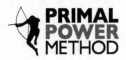

There may actually be several spots around your yard that could support a few plants. A friend of mine happily harvests a steady supply of ever-bearing strawberries from a plot just three by three feet in size.

Once you have chosen your garden plots, you will want to prepare the soil. Supporting plants that produce food will require a soil that is healthy with a balanced component of minerals along with enough organic matter to retain moisture and feed soil microorganisms, and a mix of sand and clay to ensure proper drainage.

If you have a good site in mind but it is mostly clay, then you will need to spend perhaps a full season improving the spot before you plant your garden. Pure clay can be lightened with sharp sand and even small pebbles.

If you have a spot in mind that is currently covered in grass, then here is an easy way to prepare the soil for a garden. Lay down several layers of newspapers and/or corrugated cardboard from old boxes to cover the entire area you want to turn into garden. Now cover this with generous amounts of organic materials (that is, substances that will decay) such as old hay, cow or sheep manure, straw, your own kitchen compost, bone or blood meal from reputable sources, kelp, fish meal, and so on. Choose materials that will break down completely in one season; avoid leaves (especially from oak) or twigs.

Earthworms will be attracted to this mélange of decomposing goodies and will help you along underground, digesting the grass and paper layer and loosening the soil just beneath. If there is a long dry spell while this process is underway, be sure to saturate your garden plot well at least once a week to keep the earthworms and soil organisms healthy, happy, and working for you.

At the end of the season you should be able to easily turn over this plot with a spade, further introducing the organic materials into the top layer of soil. Depending on your location, you may be ready to plant at this point, or, if the frosts of late fall or winter are approaching, you can lay down yet another layer of organic material—especially old hay, which is more nutritious than straw—and be ready to start your garden come spring.

A similar method can be done when creating raised beds, and the spaces can be simply contained with 2x4s nailed together.

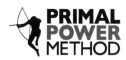

If a patio or terrace is your only outdoor space, then container gardening can be a very functional alternative. Dwarf forms of vegetables, such as cherry tomatoes and bush cucumbers can be grown quite successfully this way, and most herbs lend themselves marvelously to container plantings and are beautiful and fragrant to boot. Even dwarf fruit trees can be grown in large containers in the appropriate climates.

In the case of container gardens, do choose your soil carefully. The best choices would be your own home compost, or similar living, fertile soil from another source you trust. These plantings will benefit from frequent applications of fish emulsion and kelp to maintain nutrient and mineral levels, and to ensure the microorganisms in the soil stay healthy and confer that health to your plants.

If at all possible, try to avoid the municipal water supply when watering your garden. Chlorine, fluoride and many other contaminants in the water supply will slowly sterilize your soil and compromise the health of your garden plants (most especially those in containers). Instead, install simple rain collection barrels or buckets at your downspouts to collect rainwater for your gardening needs.

Following these methods will help ensure that your garden plants are supported by healthy, fertile soil without the inputs of synthetic fertilizers. Healthy plants will of course not require herbicides of any sort—the advantage of a small garden is that any pests that might appear can be easily spotted and picked off by you!

The rewards of harvesting and eating vegetables, fruits and herbs grown this way are golden: clean, delicious and nutritious food that you tended with pride. Share some with your neighbors and inspire them to do the same!

Creating a Compost Pile

As you gain experience with gardening, I recommend you consider creating a compost pile. Compost is decayed organic matter that provided nutrients to plants; it is one of the organic gardener's chief means of establishing a productive soil.

Nature engages in an eternal composting cycle as each year's vegetative growth returns to the soil at the end of its life: trees drop their leaves

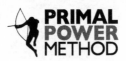

and herbaceous plants die back. This spent plant material returns the goodness that went into creating them back to the earth to be used again and again.

If you break this cycle by planting a vegetable garden and then removing and eating the produce, you must find a way to add sufficient organic material back to your garden to keep it productive.

Non-organic gardeners will use chemical or synthetic fertilizers. Like synthetic vitamins, these fertilizers will provide some nutrients, but not in the optimum form or balance for the plants. And these fertilizers will do nothing to feed and condition the soil, which is really the ultimate benefit of organic compost.

So, here's how to do it right.

The organic gardener has many options for composting at home. The first consideration is the location of the compost pile. Choose a place that is in partial to full shade, with full exposure to rain and circulating air, and good drainage. Usually a corner of the property or behind a structure such as a garage provides an adequate spot.

Depending on your location, amount of space available, propinquity of neighbors, their pets, and wildlife population, you may opt for an open, unstructured pile, or a covered container that is, at least theoretically, animal-proof. Many containers are available on the market, but while they may be adequate for the waste from your kitchen, they do not accommodate large quantities of plant material.

Simple homemade, open-topped box-like structures bounded by wood frames and wire mesh work very well and are inexpensive to build. Two or three can be constructed together so that fresh material can be added to subsequent bins as the first bins are filled, letting the first piles break down into fully decomposed compost.

With more than one box you can be filling one with new material, while another is in the process of breaking down, and you are using fully composted material from the third.

There are three basic requirements for creating a successful compost pile. The pile needs to retain the heat it generates, must receive enough air circulation to keep the process going, and enough moisture for soil

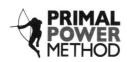

organisms to thrive while not so wet that a putrefying mess results instead of crumbly, fragrant humus (decayed vegetable or animal matter)

You can use any scrap vegetative material in the compost pile—this is a wonderful way to keep kitchen scraps out of the landfill and instead turn them into gold for your home garden, for example.

Everything except meat scraps can go into the compost pile—eggshells, cheese rinds, and moldy dairy products actually activate and feed the organisms necessary for "culturing" your compost pile, but they may be attractive to wildlife such as skunks and raccoons as well. You can decide whether this is a tolerable tradeoff or not in your location.

Tea leaves, tea sachets, and coffee grounds are a terrific addition—red worms and earthworms love them all and will happily come to work for you in your compost heap if you regularly add these.

Everything you weed from your lawn and garden can go into the compost pile—but you may want to let things like quack grass (*Agropyron repens*) fully dry out in the sun first so that you do not inadvertently introduce this pernicious weed back into your garden later.

A certain amount of dry leaves from trees can be added, but be sure to keep those layers thin, or mix them well throughout your compost. They need moisture and material higher in nitrogen to break down well. Be sure to spread out fresh grass clippings as well, since they are so moist they can become compacted into a nasty slimy mass if you fail to distribute them in the pile well.

Other good candidates for the compost heap include non-woody stalks, the leavings from your harvest of the vegetable garden, small amounts of wood shavings (avoid large amounts of saw dust or chipped bark and twigs), old straw or hay—in thin layers—cow, sheep, or other ruminant manure, already composted, and occasional small additions of poultry manure.

A caution: Do not ever use dog or cat manure or litter!

Regularly turning the material in your compost heap, or rotating the material along in successive bins, will hasten the process of decomposition, and also ensures that all layers are breaking down at the same time. Using this method you may have usable compost in as little

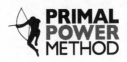

as ten weeks or so. Alternatively, you can leave the material from one year as is, and then turn it early the next spring once or twice and plan to have ready compost by planting time.

Well-rotted compost is a delightful product: crumbly with a moist, very pleasant earthy aroma. This valuable material can be spread anywhere you need it—from vegetable and fruit beds to your foundation plants and around trees. Regular application of this compost will keep soil organisms happy and prolific, with a diversity of nutrients in the soil to ultimately feed all plant life.

No wonder gardeners refer to it as black gold!

Organics in Action: A Personal and Untypical History of Family Farm Life in Last Century America

Now that you have an idea of why organic foods are so beneficial, I'd like to plant a seed in your mind about the kinds of agrarian attitudes we could be teaching the next generation of Americans.

Because so many of us grew up not steeped in a farming lifestyle – in sharp contrast no doubt to many of our grand- or great-grandparents – I have included the following story as a living example of what a return to traditional agriculture can look like.

This is a personal essay by Katherine Czapp, an independent organic famer and book editor. Her story is a wonderful example of life on a sustainable farm, and of what that kind of life can mean for and individual, a family, and a community. What follows are Katherine's words.

> I was raised on a traditional family farm in rural Michigan. My father's parents, immigrants from Eastern Europe, had purchased this farm in the 1930s with settlement money they had won from a successful suit against the coal company in Pennsylvania responsible for my grandfather's disablement in a mining accident.
>
> The dramatic change in life for my grandparents could not have been better—the return to an agrarian lifestyle entirely above

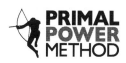

ground on the green earth under sun and rain was a continual joy to them, even in the hard times that inevitably came with working the land for one's livelihood.

My parents, although each the first in their respective families to have earned university degrees, nevertheless decided to forego careers in the city and resolved instead to return to my father's family farm to raise their children. This was in the mid 1950s, during the post World War II period when the rest of the nation was beginning to embrace with wild abandon the technologies and innovations that were the fruits of the successful U.S. military effort.

The excitement of that period of prosperity and "scientific advancement" was soon to overtake most traditional ways of life in this country, and farming was an obvious target for a complete revolutionary overhaul.

Pesticides such as DDT and the weed killer 2-4D (a major component of Agent Orange) were promoted shamelessly as safe and effective means to control bugs and weeds but their sale was really primarily intended to keep U.S. munitions factories in booming business during "peace time."

This misguided decision by the military-political cartel was in large part responsible for waging war on America's farmlands and farming families. The use of these synthetic chemicals— including petrochemical-based fertilizers—actually caused more problems than they were touted to solve, yet the trend was not to be deterred and in fact still forms the backbone of the conventional military approach to agriculture today.

The quality of food produced on soils under this perpetual chemical attack has been unequivocally documented to be substandard—the chemicals have caused degradation of soil nutrients, upset mineral balance, destroyed the soil's micro-flora, and hastened erosion, among other devastations.

Wide scale and increased mechanization was another innovative trend promoted to release the farmer from back-bending drudgery, but was really another way to dupe him into buying ever larger, more expensive machinery—leading him resolutely

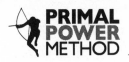

into debt as he fought ever harder to produce the enormous yields necessary to just make ends meet and pay the bankers. The deafening "get big or get out" mantra was chanted throughout the land by federal and local agricultural agencies and policy makers and this is exactly what most farmers ultimately did.

Getting big meant signing on for permanent debt, however, as farmers found the only way to keep a hair ahead of their payments was to lease more and more land in a nearly impossible bid to boost their mono-crop yields.

In the face of this compelling and nearly inescapable trend, my parents decided to neither get big nor get out, but to stay small, stay diversified, and embrace "subsistence farming." This simply means that they were replicating the lifestyle of what I would call the historical "prosperous peasant" of Europe or Asia, for example.

The modern farmer utterly relies on selling his produce to make a living—without a market he would perish, and so is ever dependent on market demand to justify his way of life. The prosperous peasant, on the other hand, raises or forages everything he and his family and all his livestock need right on his own land. Whatever surplus he sells is for his profit, but his livelihood is not dependent on market fluctuations, which he can afford to ignore when they are not favorable. As long as one has no debt and never incurs future debt, this is a most independent and satisfying way of life.

Our three-generation family did raise (organically, it goes without saying, before that term was in common use!) or forage nearly everything we ate, and we kids were introduced to a vast array of fruits and vegetables—fresh and fermented—that my mother and grandparents raised in large gardens and small orchards.

The dairy cows provided meat, milk and butter in all forms. A flock of chickens provided eggs and meat. A high-school friend of my father raised sheep and we would trade a veal calf with him when we wanted lamb. My aunt and uncle a mile down the road raised hogs, and once each fall we'd barter for a half hog along with the kidney fat to make beautiful lard.

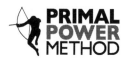

My grandparents put up sauerkraut in a hundred-gallon barrel, and my grandmother made wine from Concord grapes in her vineyard. Mushrooms appeared in the woods and fields in spring and fall, and numerous other berries and nuts were there to be gathered. Venison was an occasional treat as well.

I loved the farm life, and am grateful to this day that my parents spurned the modern trend of the time and provided this nearly vanished life for us. I enjoyed milking cows, baling hay, tending calves and chickens and gardens—responsibilities that give a child the deep pleasure of contributing to a greater good, as well as a big dose of self-reliance.

We kids worked hard, but there was always plenty of leisure to simply be a kid and watch hawks sail on the air currents, or follow a train of ants on some organized mission, or read a book, or fill your stomach from the strawberry patch, or doze off on a limb high up a maple tree.

The experience of silence—that is, apart from the pleasing cacophony of nature—is now rare. Aside from books, we did not have a great deal of material possessions, and we kids were never driven anywhere for any "amusement"—something that might be considered abuse by today's standards of child rearing.

Yet our world was a safe, secure place to us—our parents did not spend sleepless nights agonizing about bank payments or if we'd lose the farm. The actual income from the farm was so low that I won't mention it here, but it always paid for what we needed. I felt truly rich growing up, and the lesson of how to live gloriously well even in direct opposition to the prevailing definition of "successful" has served me handsomely in life.

More and more young people today are returning to a model of the small, diversified family farm as a healthy, sane way to raise their children, and a satisfying means to feed themselves and their neighbors in communities all over the country. We knew it would only be a matter of time for the wisdom of the prosperous peasant to be rediscovered by the next generation of family farms in America, and thank goodness for the return to traditional wisdom and reverence for life on this beautiful blue-green planet.

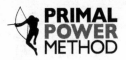

Quality Information = Quality Results

As you can see from this text, making intelligent health decisions can be a little tricky if you don't have the right information.

My goal with the Primal Power Method educational materials is to provide you with information in a way that does not overwhelm you. I have found that when individuals are given too much health and exercise information at once, they tend to become confused and don't stick to behaviors that would lead them to their health and wellness goals.

I wrote this book to complement my other wellness resources. It has one goal: to inspire you to rethink how you choose the food you and your family eat. And hopefully, to help you feel healthier and lose weight in the process.

Even though this book can stand alone, I encourage you to read my other, foundational book if you have not already done so. It's available on my website and called: *Primal Power Method: Change Your Body. Change Your Life. The Modern Caveman Lifestyle, Simplified.* It gives you a great deal of knowledge that supplements this text.

Hopefully this book has gotten you fired up about making changes in your food and lifestyle habits But I recommend taking a slow and steady, realistic approach.

The main reason I tell people to make the change in phases or steps is that it takes time to find the right stores and markets to purchase your items. You may have to join a few different CSAs before you find one that you like the best. You will also start to mix and match the stores and places you shop as you decide what products you prefer. There will be stores that specialize in certain items so you will have to shop around and see what they have to offer.

This is a lifestyle and you will be constantly learning and finding new places to shop. For example, I recently found an organic fruit and vegetable stand in a farming area where I ride my road and mountain bike. No slick advertising, just a couple of roadside signs guided you to the spot. The "market" is simply a booth set up on the honor system: you take the items you want and drop your money in a slot next to the stand.

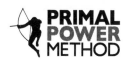

You will find as you get deeper into the world of organic foods that this type of business model is not uncommon. The farmers are busy tending to their farm and can't man the produce stand full-time. Such a system built on honor takes you back to another time when everyone trusted each other. Needless to say I will be incorporating this stand into my regular organic shopping routine.

Remember to go to our website for free articles, blogs and other health related information, at www.PrimalPowerMethod.com. I wish you luck and pleasant discoveries on your ventures into health and an organic lifestyle.

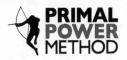

Appendix A: Organic Resources For Farmers Markets, Grass Fed Meat, CSA's, Recipes and More

EatWild
http://www.eatwild.com

• Comprehensive, accurate information about the benefits of raising animals on pasture.

• A direct link to local farms that sell all-natural, delicious, grass-fed products.

• Support for farmers who raise their livestock on pasture from birth to market and who actively promote the welfare of their animals and the health of the land.

FarmMatch
http://www.farmmatch.com

The FarmMatch mission is to re-establish fresh, local, organic and sustainable food chains around the world. We strive to empower those who believe in producing and consuming wholesome food by connecting them to one another. In this way, we aim to realize a commonly shared vision of food that sustains optimal health for our bodies and our planet.

Food Routes
http://www.foodroutes.org

The FoodRoutes Through their **Good Food** map you connect and find local farmers. Find your local food on their interactive map, listing farmers, CSAs, and local markets near you.

Eat Well Guide
http://www.eatwellguide.org

Eat Well Guide® is a free online database for finding fresh, locally grown and sustainably produced food in the United States and Canada. Listings range from stores, to farms, to restaurants, to local bakers and butchers, and visitors can search by location, keyword or category to find good food, download customized guides, or plan a trip with the innovative mapping tool **Eat Well Everywhere.**

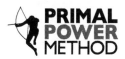

Local Harvest
http://www.localharvest.org

Local Harvest maintains a definitive and reliable living public nationwide directory of small farms, farmers markets, and other local food sources. Our search engine helps people find products from family farms, local sources of sustainably grown food, and encourages them to establish direct contact with small farms in their local area.

Farmers Market's
http://www.ams.usda.gov/farmersmarkets

USDA Directory of Farmers Market's throughout the United States

Organic Consumers Association
http://organicconsumers.org

The Organic Consumers Association is a public interest organization dedicated to promoting health justice and sustainability. A central focus of the OCA is building a healthy, equitable, and sustainable system of food production and consumption. They are a global clearinghouse for information and grassroots technical assistance.

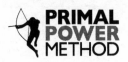

Appendix B: Bonus Report:
Real vs Fake Foods

As I noted in the introduction to this book. I would love to see us all eat organic, whole foods – but I'd much rather see everyone eating non-organic, fruits, vegetables, nuts, seeds, meats, and other whole foods that consuming the junky pseudo-foods that unfortunately dominate most American palates.

So yes, I'd love for us to all eat organic foods. But beyond that, I want everyone in America to know about the epidemic of fake, chemical-laced non-foods in our grocery stores, pantries, and lives. That's what this section is about.

We all need to ask ourselves: What are we putting in our bodies on a daily basis and why is it making us so sick?

For example, who couldn't resist a strawberry shake and some chicken nuggets? I mean, they are prepared from strawberries and chicken, right?

Not exactly. Here's the full ingredient list for a Chicken McNugget (from McDonalds' website):

> White boneless chicken, water, food starch – modified, salt, seasoning (autolyzed yeast extract, salt, wheat starch, natural flavoring (botanical source), safflower oil, dextrose, citric acid, rosemary), sodium phosphates, seasoning (canola oil, mono- and diglycerides, extractives of rosemary). Battered and breaded with: water, enriched flour (bleached wheat flour, niacin, reduced iron, thiamin mononitrate, riboflavin, folic acid), yellow corn flour, food starch –modified, salt, leavening (baking soda, sodium acid pyrophosphate, sodium aluminum phosphate, monocalcium phosphate, calcium lactate), spices, wheat starch, whey, corn starch. Prepared in vegetable oil (canola oil, corn oil, soybean oil, hydrogenated soybean oil with TBHQ and citric acid added to preserve freshness). Dimethylpolysiloxane added as an antifoaming agent.

Do you find this as gross and un-food-like as I do?

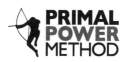

But it gets worse. The "white boneless chicken" as listed above is made up of pulverized chicken skin and mechanically reclaimed meat. Why is that suboptimal? Mechanically reclaimed meat is a paste-like meat product produced by forcing beef, pork or chicken bones, with any attached edible meat, through a sieve or similar device under high pressure. This process separates the bone from the "edible" meat tissue.

Surprisingly, the reclaimed meat only accounts for about half of an actual McNugget. The remaining 50 percent of the food item is made up in large part by corn derivatives, sugars, leavening agents and other completely synthetic ingredients.

Here are some of the other uses and side effects of various McNugget ingredients:

> *Dimethylpolysiloxane:* This is an anti-foaming agent: a chemical added during a heating process to reduce the formation of surface foam. (Foaming chicken for lunch? Any takers?) It's made of silicone and also used in Silly Putty and cosmetics.

> *Tertiary butylhydroquinone (TBHQ):* This chemical preservative is a form of butane (also known as lighter fluid). One gram of TBHQ can cause nausea, vomiting, ringing in the ears, delirium, a sense of suffocation, and physical collapse.

(Here's where one of the principles of the Primal Power Method – outlined in the first chapter of this book – really applies: Keep it simple. This applies to ingredient lists: if you can't pronounce it or recognize it, don't eat it!)

Well, we just can't have those nuggets without something to wash them down, so below are some of the ingredients (many of which are likely unrecognizable as food) you may find in the modern fast food strawberry shake:

> Milkfat and nonfat milk, sugar, sweet whey, high-fructose corn syrup, guar gum, monoglycerides and diglycerides, cellulose gum, sodium phosphate, carrageenan, citric acid, E129 and artificial strawberry flavor.

And what does that seemingly simple and innocent ingredient called "artificial strawberry flavor" really contain?

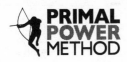

Just these few yummy chemicals: amyl acetate, amyl butyrate, amyl valerate, anethol, anisyl formate, benzyl acetate, benzyl isobutyrate, butyric acid, cinnamyl isobutyrate, cinnamyl valerate, cognac essential oil, diacetyl, dipropyl ketone, ethyl butyrate, ethyl cinnamate, ethyl heptanoate, ethyl heptylate, ethyl lactate, ethyl methylphenylglycidate, ethyl nitrate, ethyl propionate, ethyl valerate, heliotropin, hydroxyphrenyl-2-butanone (10% solution in alcohol), ionone, isobutyl anthranilate, isobutyl butyrate, lemon essential oil, maltol, 4-methylacetophenone, methyl anthranilate, methyl benzoate, methyl cinnamate, methyl heptine carbonate, methyl naphthyl ketone, methyl salicylate, mint essential oil, neroli essential oil, nerolin, neryl isobutyrate, orris butter, phenethyl alcohol, rose, rum ether, undecalactone, vanillin and solvent.

Now let's compare this mad scientist's laboratory brew with the ingredients of healthy, or shall we say, organic chicken nuggets and a strawberry shake made in a home kitchen:

Chicken Nugget:

• Meat from whole, free-ranging, happy chickens raised without steroids, GMO feed, and antibiotics.

• Minimally processed nut-based or other type of gluten free flour.

• Whole herbs, spices and seasonings, perhaps from your own windowsill garden.

• Organic eggs from the above chickens for the batter.

• Virgin coconut oil.

Strawberry Shake:

• Strawberries fresh from the farm, grown without herbicides or synthetic fertilizers.

• Whole organic milk from free range, grass fed cows.

• Ice.

Hmmm, just a little bit of a difference!

And as someone who has made chicken nuggets and a strawberry shake from all (real) organic ingredients, I can attest that there is absolutely no comparison in taste or quality.

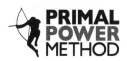

A similar comparison may be drawn between real butter and its fake-foods pseudo-clone: margarine.

Today's margarine typically contains some combination of the following chemical components: sterol esters, genetically modified liquid soybean oil, liquid canola oil, hydrogenated soybean oil, partially hydrogenated soybean oil, soy lecithin, vegetable mono and diglycerides, potassium sorbate, calcium disodium EDTA, artificial flavors and synthetic vitamins.

Remember, if it doesn't sound like food, it isn't food.

Take the example of one of the ingredients in many brands of margarine, calcium disodium EDTA. It is a pharmaceutical-grade chelating agent (a chemical substance capable of bonding securely to minute particles of metal called ions). It is designed to make certain trace metals inactive (such as nickel oxide used in the manufacture of margarine).

It sounds awful, but it gets worse.

Margarine is naturally grey in color – this color is bleached with chemical additives. Dyes and strong flavors are then added to help it physically masquerade as butter. The final mixture is compressed and packaged and sold as a "magical" health food, if you can stomach it!

Now, consider the ingredients in organic butter: cream from real milk, and sometimes sea salt. Amazingly, butter has been demonized for over a century, yet so often health lies in simplicity and authenticity.

Bottom line: Skip the margarine and faux-butter substitutes, and just have some organic, natural butter instead.

Let me say it plainly: Those of you who have watched movies such as *Farmageddon, Food, Inc.*, or *Supersize Me* know what I'm talking about when it comes to the differences between our mass produced "food products" and real food from organic farms. For those of you who have not watched any of the above movies/documentaries I highly recommend you do so as the visual representations of our modern monolithic agricultural industry—usually kept far away from public scrutiny—are truly shocking.

What follows is a summary of all of the chemical nonsense that makes its way onto the dinner plates of most Americans. Please read, learn, and avoid these unhealthy food choices as much as is humanly possible.

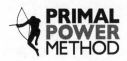

Preservatives, Additives, and Food Processing: A Huge Hidden Danger

Our ancestors used natural food preservation ingredients and techniques, including salt, fermentation or drying foods in the sun. Modern processing has deviated drastically from these simple practices toward more complicated, chemical-based methods.

Here's what it boils down to: Processed foods typically contain a chemical soup of additives and preservatives thrown in to "improve" the shelf-life, appearance, and flavor of what was once a recognizable food. As if you needed more reasons to avoid over-processed, unhealthy, fattening pseudo-foods!

Today, food companies use nearly six thousand additives and chemicals to process the products we eat. Many of these chemicals will have a devastating effect on our health. What follows is an overview of the types of chemicals that most of us eat on a daily basis. As you'll see, it's enough to make you – literally – sick.

The Truth about Processed Food

When we talk about foods you should not eat, we are almost always talking about processed foods. It's important to know the facts about these sometimes not-so-obviously junk foods… a truth that the food industry and the government often will not provide.

Today's grocery stores are loaded with heavily processed items that should not even be categorized as food. Manufacturers argue that such items give consumers what they want: food that is fast, cheap, and easy to prepare.

However, industrial food processing destroys essential nutrients and makes these products difficult to digest. It also uses products and processes that nearly guarantee a negative impact on your long-term health. These include ingredients like sugar, white flour, processed and hydrogenated oils, additives, synthetic vitamins, and plenty of empty calories, as well as harsh and damaging processing techniques such as the extrusion of grains and hexane extraction of so-called edible oils.

This section will discuss some of these issues in detail and elucidate just why unadulterated, as-found-in-nature organic food choices are always your best bet.

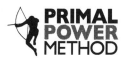

Three Types of Food Culprits

There are three categories of food products on the commercial mass market today: processed food, junk food, and fake food.

Processed food is made from real (natural) food that has been put through devitalizing processes to make it (supposedly) more appealing, and infused with chemicals and preservatives to enhance its shelf life. Canned and bottled tea, jam, hot dogs, most kinds of beef jerky, and low-fat yogurt with sugar or aspartame are a few examples.

Junk foods are even worse, since they contain very little real food. They're made from devitalized processed food, hydrogenated fats, chemicals and preservatives, and include anything made with refined white flour (including home-made baked goods). Canned breakfast drinks, sugary cereals, doughnuts, foods tendered at drive-through establishments and sodas and soft drinks are other examples.

Fake foods are made primarily from chemicals, and often contain gums and sugar fillers. Examples include "bacon bits," many bottled salad dressings, dehydrated soups, and instant coffee. These appalling non-foods take more energy for your body to process, neutralize, and eliminate than they contain in nutritional value. They leave your body sluggish and depleted.

As those of you have read other Primal Power books and reports know, American health statistics are grim. The U.S. ranks amongst the lowest of all industrialized nations in terms of life expectancy.

Americans consume over a third of their calories through junk foods and spend more than 120 billion dollars on fast foods per year. The list of appalling concoctions we mindlessly ingest in the name of dubious nourishment is long. What are these dietary culprits comprised of? What makes them so toxic? Most importantly, what are they doing to our bodies? Read on to find out.

Preservatives: Nitrates and Nitrites, Sulfites, Benzoic Acid, and Antioxidants

Preservatives are added to foods to help prevent spoilage. They come in many varieties.

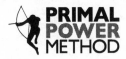

Nitrates and Nitrites

Nitrates are naturally occurring compounds that are created when plants break down nitrogen during photosynthesis (the chemical process that allows plants to store solar energy as sugar). When nitrates come in contact with certain bacteria, they break down into nitrites. Both are used to preserve meats such as bacon and ham and are known to cause vomiting, nausea, and headaches in some people.

When you read that a meat (such as ham) has been "cured," it means that it has been preserved with artificial nitrates and nitrites. Conventional food manufacturers use synthetic sodium nitrite to cure processed meat products.

According to the third edition of the National Academy of Science's Food Chemical Codex – a document that lists internationally recognized purity and identity standards of food ingredients – food-grade sodium nitrite is permitted to contain residual heavy metals, arsenic, and lead.

Sodium nitrite is capable of being converted to nitrous acid when ingested by humans. Even though animal testing shows that nitrous acid causes high rates of cancer, sodium nitrate is still in use today, and is the "meat-curing" industry standard for most food manufacturers.

"Uncured" meats also contain nitrates and nitrites. However, these are naturally-occurring. Most natural or organic meat companies use celery powder and sea salt as a preservative in place of synthetic sodium nitrate. The celery powder and sea salt react with added lactic acid starter culture and convert into natural nitrites to cure natural meats such as organic bacon or ham.

The easiest way to tell if the meat you are purchasing contains natural or chemical nitrates and/or nitrites is to look for on the label for "no nitrites or nitrates added" or "no nitrates/nitrites other than naturally occurring." Natural nitrates/nitrites are the healthier choice since they have not been found to cause cancer.

Remember: The USDA defines an uncured product as one that has been preserved without the use of synthetic sodium nitrite. Look for "no nitrites or nitrates added" or the food label and choose organic, naturally cured meats.

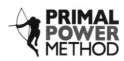

Sulfites

Sulfites are commonly used to prevent fungal spoilage and the browning of peeled fruits and vegetables. Sulfites are added to many processed foods and beverages as preservatives.

Sulfites are safe for most people. However, the FDA estimates that one out of 100 people is sensitive to sulfites and that approximately five percent of asthma sufferers may have an adverse reaction to sulfites.

You may develop an allergy to sulfites at any point in life. The most common symptom is difficulty breathing. Allergic responses include chest tightness, dizziness, nausea, cramps, hives, and wheezing.

According to the Food Marketing Institute, the food industry uses six sulfiting agents. **If any of these ingredients is on a food label, it means the product contains sulfites and should be avoided:**

- Sulfur dioxide
- Sodium sulfite
- Sodium bisulfite
- Potassium bisulfite
- Sodium metabisulfite
- Potassium metabisulfite

Benzoic Acid

Benzoic acid (also known as sodium benzoate) is added to margarine, fruit juices, and carbonated beverages. There have been some health concerns regarding the combination of sodium benzoate and ascorbic acid (vitamin C), most commonly found in fruit juices and fruit-flavored soft drinks. When the two are mixed, they can form the chemical benzene, which is carcinogenic.

Antioxidants

Today, almost every type of processed food contains antioxidant preservatives. These help prevent fatty foods from spoiling when exposed to oxygen.

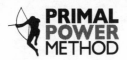

Two of the most controversial and frequently used chemical antioxidants are BHT (butylated hydroxytoluene) and BHA (butylated hydroxyanisole). BHT and BHA consumption has been associated with alarming negative health effects in animal studies – so much so that a number of countries have greatly restricted their use (although, sadly, this is not the case in America).

BHA is added to butter, meats, cereals, chewing gum, baked goods, snack foods, dehydrated potatoes and beer. It is also found in animal feed, food packaging, cosmetics, rubber products and petroleum products. BHT is added directly to shortening, cereals, and other foods containing fats and oils.

Some people have difficulty metabolizing BHT and BHA. These difficulties are thought to lead to hyperactivity and other health and behavioral problems. These chemicals can also cause allergic reactions, may contribute to the development of tumors and cancer, and may be toxic to the nervous system and liver.

Despite these findings, the use of BHT and BHA as preservatives in the food industry has increased, rather than decreased, in America.

Additives: Thickeners, Emulsifiers and Stabilizers, Artificial Colors, and Artificial Flavors

Thickeners, Emulsifiers and Stabilizers

Thickeners, emulsifiers and stabilizers are additives that alter the texture of foods. Emulsifiers, for example, prevent ingredients from separating into unappealing globs in products such as mayonnaise and ice cream.

Propylene glycol is an example of a synthetic solvent used as an emulsifier in foods. It's also a first cousin to anti-freeze. Although it's toxic to the skin and sensory organs and is considered to be a brain-damaging neurotoxin, the FDA has deemed it "generally recognized as safe" (GRAS).

A "Generally Recognized as Safe" (GRAS) rating is given to a substance that is generally recognized, among qualified experts, as "safe" under the conditions of its intended use, or unless the use of the substance is otherwise excluded from the definition of a food additive.

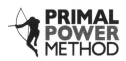

In my view, in the real world a GRAS rating doesn't mean much. Just eat natural, unprocessed foods!

> **Generally Recognized as Safe (GRAS)**
>
> "GRAS" is an acronym for the phrase Generally Recognized As Safe. Under sections 201(s) and 409 of the Federal Food, Drug, and Cosmetic Act any substance that is intentionally added to food is a food additive and is subject to pre-market review and approval by the Federal Drug Administration (the FDA).
>
> In my opinion, GRAS standards are useless since they do not truly differentiate between ingredients that are truly dangerous (or not) to our health. Plus, many GRAS ingredients are unnatural chemical food additives, which just have no place in a quest for optimal human health.

In my view, in the real world a GRAS rating doesn't mean much. Just eat natural, unprocessed foods!

Artificial Colors

Every year, the American food industry adds three thousand tons of artificial coloring to the foods we eat.

Many foods and beverages are routinely altered, including popcorn, hot dogs, jellies, jellybeans, carbonated beverages, butter, margarine, maraschino cherries, canned strawberries and peas, and the colors of the skins of fresh oranges and potatoes.

Even chicken feed on large-scale egg farms is artificially colored so that chickens will lay golden-yolked eggs – similar to those honestly laid by their free-ranging and organically raised counterparts who enjoy green vegetation and sunshine.

For now, it's sufficient for you to know that many coloring agents are derived from coal tar (that is, they are petroleum products), and nearly all are synthetic. Artificial colors have also been linked to allergies, asthma and hyperactivity.

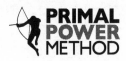

Outside of America, these substances are recognized as dangerous. Norway, for example, maintains a total ban on all products containing coal tar. But although some cancer-linked artificial food dyes have been banned in this country, many other artificial colors are still in use today.

Artificial Flavors

Flavorings are the most common type of food additive.There are over 2,000 natural and artificial flavors in use today.

Once again, the ingredients of the artificial strawberry flavor used in some popular fast food restaurants' strawberry milk shakes are listed below. After reading this list, I can almost guarantee you will never look at a milkshake in the same way again:

> Amyl acetate, amyl butyrate, amyl valerate, anethol, anisyl formate, benzyl acetate, benzyl isobutyrate, butyric acid, cinnamyl isobutyrate, cinnamyl valerate, cognac essential oil, diacetyl, dipropyl ketone, ethyl butyrate, ethyl cinnamate, ethyl heptanoate, ethyl heptylate, ethyl lactate, ethyl methylphenylglycidate, ethyl nitrate, ethyl propionate, ethyl valerate, heliotropin, hydroxyphrenyl-2-butanone (10% solution in alcohol), ionone, isobutyl anthranilate, isobutyl butyrate, lemon essential oil, maltol, 4-methylacetophenone, methyl anthranilate, methyl benzoate, methyl cinnamate, methyl heptine carbonate, methyl naphthyl ketone, methyl salicylate, mint essential oil, neroli essential oil, nerolin, neryl isobutyrate, orris butter, phenethyl alcohol, rose, rum ether, undecalactone, vanillin and solvent.

Artificial flavors have been linked to allergic and behavioral reactions, yet these ingredients are not required to be listed on food product labels in detail as they're Generally Recognized as Safe (GRAS) by the FDA. What you may see on a food label instead are ambiguous terms like "artificial flavor" which could mean almost anything.

According to the GRAS standards, the precise ingredients of this popular fast food strawberry shake don't have to be listed anywhere. For those of us who read food labels religiously, this is truly scary, since you may think you are choosing a food item with few artificial ingredients, but in actuality are getting an alphabet soup of toxic garbage.

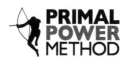

Monosodium glutamate (MSG) is a common and popular **flavor-enhancer**. It has been found to cause damage in laboratory mice and has been banned from use in baby foods, yet is still used in numerous other food products. It can cause allergic and behavioral reactions such as headaches, dizziness, chest pains, depression and mood swings, and is also a possible neurotoxin (a chemical that damages or destroys nerve tissue).

A Note on "Natural" Flavors and Colors

In a bid for health, you may have heretofore bypassed artificial colors and flavors in favor of "natural" alternatives listed on food labels. Here is what I want you to know about these ingredients.

"Natural flavors" can be made from just about anything – from the cells of yeast extract to cattle waste byproducts. Some reports suggest that the ingredients of so-called natural colors have been known to contain products as unlikely as monkey intestines; others note that certain artificial flavors are comprised of ingredients as unappealing as minced cat.

This doesn't mean that all natural flavors are bad, but when you see the word "natural" on a label you should take it with a grain of salt and a good deal of skepticism. In today's world of food additives, the definition of "natural flavors" is cast with an exceedingly wide and liberal net.

To wit, the aforementioned ground-up cat meat is natural... but I'm not too sure I want it as an additive in the foods I eat.

The Processes behind Processed Foods: Bleaching, Refining, Extrusion, Irradiation, and Packaging

Nearly six thousand chemicals and additives are used in everyday foods. But on top of this, food-preserving processes have changed beyond recognition. In the past, natural foods were preserved with techniques such as lacto-fermentation, vinegar, salt and the drying effects of sunshine. Today's preservation techniques strip the nutrients from many processed foods, leaving them with little or no nutritional value.

Worse, foods are deliberately tampered with to make them more palatable and stimulate your desire to continually consume them. Plus, the health effects of eating foods treated by certain processing methods, such as irradiation, a very controversial technique, are not yet known.

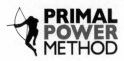

As author Marion Nestlé writes in *What to Eat:* "Heavy processing does three things to foods: diminishes the nutritional value of the basic ingredients; adds calories from fats, and sugars; and disguises the loss of taste and texture with salt, artificial colors, flavors, and other additives."

This section will discuss more details of the dangers of food processing techniques, including bleaching, refining, extrusion, irradiation and food packaging.

Bleaching

Changing whole grain wheat into the white flour commonly used in baked goods involves a process called bleaching. This method transforms the naturally yellowish or grey tinge of freshly milled flour into a "cleaner looking" white, ostensibly to make it more appealing to consumers. Various bleaching agents may be used, including nitrogen oxide, chlorine, chloride, nitrosyl and benzoyl peroxide mixed with a variety of chemical salts.

However, these bleaching agents are not without health dangers. For example, chlorine oxide (chlorine gas) catalyzes a chemical reaction in the body that destroys beta (insulin-creating) cells in the pancreas and is now linked to diabetes. The Environmental Protection Agency (EPA) defines chlorine gas as a flour-bleaching, aging and oxidizing agent that is also a powerful irritant, dangerous to inhale, and lethal.

These toxic effects are common knowledge in the scientific community. Despite widespread awareness of its deleterious effects, the FDA still allows companies to use chlorine oxide in processed foods.

Refining

Refined flour is an ingredient in many food products. Nevertheless, it is unhealthy. This is because the process of refining the flour removes many of the grain's most nutritious elements, leaving only a starchy, vitamin-stripped version of a previously robust grain for you to eat.

To create refined flour, whole (healthy) grains are milled so that the natural brown husk (bran) of the grain as well as its oily germ are stripped away.

This leaves only a white, refined starch that is used to make white bread, pasta, cookies, baked goods and numerous other junk foods. The now-discarded fibrous husk would normally slow down the digestion of the

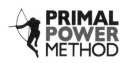

wheat product. Without it, flour's refined starches are quickly broken down into sugar and are immediately absorbed into the bloodstream. This causes blood-glucose levels to rise. Not surprisingly, a diet heavy in refined-flour-based foods has been linked to obesity.

In contrast, whole grains (such as whole grain breads, whole grain cereals, brown rice and barley) all retain the layer of bran that surrounds the grain's inner starches. Thus whole grain products, when eaten, are absorbed into the bloodstream more slowly than refined starches. This slows sugar absorption in the intestine and reduces the risk of obesity.

The Costs of Being Refined

Refining flour takes a healthy, natural whole food and turns it into empty carbs. The nutritional toll refinement takes is high.

Unsaturated fatty acids, which are healthy and high in food value, are also lost during the milling of refined flours. Half of the vitamin E of the original whole grain is destroyed when wheat germ and bran are removed during processing. Refining wheat into white flour also removes between 50 to 93 percent of the whole grain's vitamins and minerals including magnesium, zinc, chromium, manganese and cobalt.

Other casualties of the refinement process include approximately 50 percent of a whole grain's calcium, 70 percent of its phosphorus, 80 percent of its iron, 50 percent of its potassium, 65 percent of its copper, 80 percent of its thiamin (vitamin B1), 60 percent of its riboflavin (vitamin B2), 75 percent of its niacin (vitamin B3), 50 percent of its pantothenic acid (vitamin B5), and about 50 percent of its pyridoxine (vitamin B6).

Similarly, when sugar cane is refined into white sugar, 99 percent of its magnesium and 93 percent of its chromium are depleted. Polishing rice removes 75 percent of its zinc and chromium. Refined table salt has also had most of its trace minerals removed during processing.

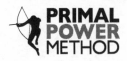
PRIMAL
POWER
METHOD

Chemicals in Bread

Refined flour is an unhealthy component of breads, pastries, and other processed foods. However, concerns with such foods go beyond the shortcomings of the flour itself, since many unhealthy chemicals and additives are added to flour-based foods. Most of the chemicals added to white flour, and therefore white breads, are not healthy and can potentially cause harm.

Take the case of potassium bromate, which is often added to white flour as an "improver" to strengthen the resultant dough and allow it to rise when baked. Unfortunately, potassium bromate is also a carcinogen (i.e., a substance known to cause cancer).

Potassium bromate has been banned from use in food products in Europe, Canada and some other countries. It was banned in Sri Lanka in 2001 and China in 2005. It is also banned in Nigeria, Brazil, and Peru.

In the United States the FDA sanctioned the use of bromate prior to the adoption of the 1958 Delaney clause of the Food, Drug, and Cosmetic Act (which bans carcinogenic substances). This pre-existence makes it more difficult to ban now. Instead, since 1991 the FDA has merely urged bakers to voluntarily stop using it. In California a warning label is required when bromated flour is used.

If potassium bromate is not overtly listed on the product label, you will find it disguised as "enriched flour" or "dough conditioner."

Another chemical, alloxan, is added to white flour to make it appear "clean" to the consumer. Alloxan also destroys beta cells (cells that make and release insulin) that are located in the pancreas. This chemical is often given to laboratory rats to induce diabetes. Yet despite the connection between alloxan and type 2 diabetes, the Food and Drug Administration (FDA) still allows its use in everyday foods.

Scientists have known of the alloxan-diabetes connection for years. Researchers who study diabetes commonly use the chemical to induce the disorder in lab animals. In that sense, giving alloxan to an animal is similar to injecting that animal with a deadly virus, since both alloxan and the virus are being used specifically to cause illness!

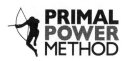

Extrusion

Dry breakfast cereals are produced via a process called extrusion. A slurry of grains is put into a machine called an extruder, which forces them out of a hole at a high pressure and temperature that deform the protein molecules within the grains. Regular consumption of these denatured grain proteins can wreak havoc on the digestive system.

Next, a blade slices off each flake or shape, which is then sprayed with a coating of oil and sugar that helps the cereal repel milk and maintain its crunchy texture.

Extruding strips grains of nutrients, such as vitamins and fatty acids. Therefore prior to the extrusion process, manufacturers may attempt to "fortify" refined grains with added vitamins (chemical-derived vitamins, which are far different from the ones naturally found in food). However, extruding can destroy even the added vitamins.

All cold, boxed cereals are made this way, even the organic ones sold in health food stores. Avoid them.

By virtue of the extrusion process, the shelf life of cold cereals is greatly extended, thus saving the manufacturers and retailers untold sums of money by reducing spoilage. These processes are designed to cut production costs, not to make nutritious food.

Needless to say I no longer consume any cereal products as they are mostly devoid of nutrients and chock full of unhealthy chemical vitamin derivatives.

Irradiation

Irradiation is a process based on the use of gamma radiation or x-rays (both of which are forms of electromagnetic radiation). Irradiation kills mold, bacteria, viruses and parasites on food.

However, there are unhealthy trade-offs: Test animals fed a diet of irradiated wheat developed increased chromosomal abnormalities. There have also been unexplained stillbirths in the offspring of test rats fed a diet of irradiated food.

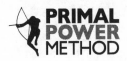

The term "irradiation" is so unpleasant to consumers that food companies use euphemisms such as "Cold Pasteurization" and "Picowaved For Your Protection" to describe irradiated food – thus avoiding an unpopular term with doomsday associations that could potentially hurt sales.

Irradiated Food: Not So Clean?

As I was researching this food processing technique, an author made the point that companies that irradiate their food products seem to be less thorough in other basic areas of hygiene.

They often act as though the irradiation process takes care of the possible risk of your food containing contaminants, such as fecal matter, and are negligent in other routine methods of cleaning (like simple washing).

It appears that more fecal matter is making its way into our foods. Irradiated or not, I'm sure you'd prefer that fecal matter stay out of your food supply!

Packaging

When it comes to your health, the materials used to coat and package foods are also suspect. Here are some examples:

Wax: The protective wax on produce such as cucumbers, peppers and apples may contain allergy-triggers such as pesticides, fungicide sprays, or animal byproducts.

Wrappers: The plastic (vinyl chloride) found in some food wrappers is considered carcinogenic, and has been linked to immune reactions and "lung shock." The latter condition (also known as Adult Respiratory Distress Syndrome) is a serious health concern characterized by respiratory failure that usually requires hospitalization.

Containers: Dioxins are chemical byproducts of the whitening process that is used to color food containers. Sadly, they have also raised health concerns. It has been reported, for example, that certain ice creams contain high levels of dioxins, reportedly leaked into the product through the whitening agents used in ice cream containers.

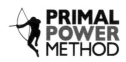

As known carcinogens, dioxins are associated with genetic and reproductive defects and learning disabilities. Dioxin exposure is a possible cause of other health conditions such as endometriosis (a painful condition that can result in fertility problems and/or necessitate a hysterectomy) as well as chronic pelvic pain.

Avoiding the Problem

I think now the picture of where our modern food processing industry fits into our health crisis in America is becoming clearer.

The best way to avoid these problems is to eat whole, organic foods, as they are found in nature. Always pay attention to the food you buy, especially if it has been refined or processed in any way.

Remember, most processed food ingredients have nothing to do with nutrition and everything to do with increasing food sales by keeping addicted, depleted consumers coming back for more. Why else would a grocery store stock tens of thousands of items? You could spend your entire existence in nature and only consume a hundred different foods if you were lucky; there would be no chance of eating thousands of different types of foods, this I guarantee.

Good Food Gone Bad

The processed food industry, which replaced healthy foods with pseudo- and junk-food imposters, tells us their "improved" products will make us healthier. But interestingly, the opposite is actually true. These concoctions make us sicker and fatter while ensuring that the industry stockholders become richer.

I'm sure after reviewing these preceding sections you get the idea: organic, organic, organic!

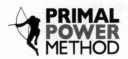

Sources

Abend, Lisa. "How Cows (Grass-Fed Only) Could Save the Planet." *Time.* 25 JAN 2010. Web. JULY 17 2012.

Badgley, Catherine, et al. "Renewable Agriculture and Food Systems." *Cambridge University Press* 22 (2007): 86-108.

Baginski, Caren. "1 Million Americans tell FDA to label genetically engineered food." *Newhope360.* 27 March 2012. Web. 29 March 2012.

Bareuther, Carol. "Mission Organic 2010: Healthy People, Healthy Planet." *Today's Dietitian* 10.4 (2008): 30.

Baulk, E., et al. "Effects of Soy on Health Outcomes." *Ahrq.* Agency for Healthcare Research and Quality. Web. 15 NOV 2010.

Bernstein and Willet. "Trends in 24-h urinary sodium excretion in the United States, 1957-2003: a systematic review." *American Journal of Clinical Nutrition* 92.5 (2010): 1172-1180.

"Biomedicine: The (Political) Science of Salt." The American Association for the Advancement of Science 281.5379 (Aug 1998): 898-907.

Burke, Cindy. *To Buy or Not to Buy Organic: What You Need to Know to Choose the Healthiest Safest, Most Earth-Friendly Food* (New York: Marlowe & Company, 2007).

Butcher, Mavis. "Genetically Modified Food: GM Food List and Information." *Disabled-world.* 22 SEP 2009. Web. 17 June 2012.

Butter is Better. Washington DC: Weston A. Price Foundation, 2010.

Carson, Rachael. *Silent Spring* (New York: Houghton Mifflin Company, 2002).

Certified Naturally Grown. "Frequently Asked Questions." *Naturallygrown.* Web. 20 JULY 2012.

Cheadle, A, et al. "Community-level comparisons between the grocery store environment and individual dietary practices." *Journal of Preventative Medicine* 20 (1991): 250-261.

Cornucopia Institute. "Cereal Crimes: How "Natural" Claims Deceive Consumers and Undermine the Organic Label – A Look Down the Cereal and Granola Aisle." *Cornucopia Institute Report* (October 2011).

Daniel, Kaayla. "Bad News for the Soy Industry." *Westonaprice.* 27 FEB 2009. Web. 15 NOV 2010.

Daniel, Kayla. *The Whole Soy Story* (Washington DC: New Trends Publishing, 2005).

Daniel, Kaayla. "What is Edamame? And Other Questions About Green Vegetable Soybeans." *Westonaprice.* 21 SEP 2010. Web. 16 NOV 2010.

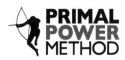

Dhiman, T. et al. "Conjugated linoleic acid content of milk from cows fed different diets." *Journal of Dairy Science* 82.10 (1999): 2146-2156.

Eaton, S. Boyd. "The ancestral human diet: what was it and should it be a paradigm for contemporary nutrition?". *Proceedings of the Nutrition Society* 65.1 (2006): 1-6.

Environmental Working Group. "Body burden: The pollution in newborns." *Ewg.* 14 JULY 2005. Web. 7 JULY 2012.

Environmental Working Group. "EWG's 2012 Shopper's Guide to Pesticides in Produce." *Ewg.* Web. 7 JULY 2012.

Ettinger, Jill. "DOA: Cows Fed GMO Corn Died, Syngeta Faces Criminal Charges." *Organicauthority.* 21 JUNE 2012. Web. 24 JUNE 2012.

Fang, Carolyn Y., et al. "Correlates of Soy Food Consumption in Women at Increased Risk for Breast Cancer." *Journal of the American Dietetic Association* 105.10 (2005): 1552-1558.

Food and Water Watch. "Genetically Engineered Food: An Overview." *Foodandwaterwatch.* 29 SEPT 2011. Web. 29 March 2011.

Food and Water Watch. "Factory Farms." *Foodandwaterwatch.* Web. 16 APRIL 2012.

Food and Water Watch. "They Eat What?." *Foodandwaterwatch.* 8 AUG 2008. Web. 16 APRIL 2012.

Gibbs, Shawn, et al. "Airborne antibiotic resistant and nonresistant bacteria and fungi recovered from two swine herd confined animal feeding operations." *Journal of Occupational and Environmental Hygiene* 1.11 (2004): 699-706.

Glanz, Karen, et al. "Retail Grocery Store Marketing Strategies and Obesity: An Integrative Review." *American Journal of Preventative Medicine* 42.5 (2012): 503-512.

Global Food Security. "Modern agriculture and food security – a history." *Foodsecurity.* Web. 19 MAY 2012.

Green, Christopher, et al. "Bacterial plume emanating from the air surrounding swine confinement." *Journal of Occupational and Environmental Hygiene* 3.1 (2006): 9-15.

Green Right Now. "Ten Reasons to buy local food." *Greenrightnow.* Web. 18 JULY 2012.

Gore, Suzanne. "What You Should Know About Organic Foods." *Journal of Renal Nutrition* 18.4 (2008): 13-15.

Halweil, Brian. "Still No Free Lunch: Nutrient Levels in U.S. food supply eroded by pursuit of high yields." *Organic-center.* SEPT 2007. Web. 7 JULY 2012.

Hartman Group. "Beyond Organic and Natural: Resolving Confusion in Marketing Foods and Beverages." *Hartmen-group.* 22 FEB 2010. Web. 22 MAY 2012.

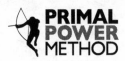

"Health Benefits of Milk." *Organicfacts*. Web. 23 NOV 2010.

Hebeisen, F. et al. "Increased concentrations of omega-3 fatty acids in milk and platelet rich plasma of grass-fed cows." *International Journal for Vitamin and Nutrition Research* 63 (1993): 229-233.

HelpGuide. "Understanding Organic Food Labels, Benefits, and Claims." *Helpguide*. Web. 23 JUNE 2012.

Henkel, J. "Soy. Health claims for soy protein, questions about other components." *FDA Consum* 34.3 (2000): 13-20.

"History of Soybeans." *Soya*. Web. 15 NOV 2010.

Holland, Laurence and David Ewalt. "How Americans Make And Spend Their Money." *Forbes*. 19 JULY 2006. Web. 11 May 2012.

Holt-Gimenez, E. "A Study of 1,804 organic farms in Central America hit my Hurricane Mitch." *Panna*. (2000) Web. 18 JULY 2012.

Hooper L., et al. "Systematic review of long term effects of advice to reduce dietary salt in adults." *British Medical Journal* 325.7365 (2002): 628.

Hyman, Mark. "Soy Alert." *Wise Traditions*. 11.3 (2010): 75-80.

Inagami, Sanae, et al. "Your Are Where You Shop: Grocery Store Locations, Weight, and Neighborhoods." *American Journal of Preventative Medicine* 31.1 (2006): 10-17.

Kaneshiro, Neil. "Trans Fatty Acids." *Nlmnih*. 2 JULY 2009. Web. 26 OCT 2010.

Kurlansky, Mark. Salt: *A World History* (New York: Penguin, 2003).

Local Harvest. "Community Supported Agriculture." *Localharvest*. Web. 18 JULY 2012.

Lotter, Donald. "Organic Agriculture." *Journal of Sustainable Agriculture* 21.4 (2003): 59-128.

Maeder, P, et al. "Soil Fertility and Biodiversity in Organic Farming." *Science* 296 (2002): 1694-1697.

Martin, N., et al. "Results from raw milk microbiological tests do not predict the shelf-life performance of commercially pasteurized fluid milk." *Journal of Dairy Science* 94.3 (2011): 1211-1222.

Mayo Clinic. "Free range and other meat and poultry terms." *Mayoclinic*. Web 23 JUNE 2012.

Mayo Clinic Staff. "Organic foods: Are they safer? More nutritious?" *Mayoclinic*. Web. 14 JULY 2012.

Mercola, Joseph D.O. "Add This Seasoning to your Food Daily – Despite What your Doctor Says." 20 SEP 2011. Web. 23 SEP 2011.

Mercola, Joseph. "Take Heed – Nearly Every Processed Food You Eat is Contaminated with the Material." *Mercola*. 29 NOV 2011. Web. 29 MARCH 2012.

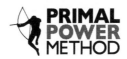

Mercola, Joseph. "This Food Knowingly Causes Cancer in Rats – Are You Eating it?" *Mercola.* 5 OCT 2011. Web. 29 MARCH 2012.

Michael, Paul. "The Dirty Secrets of Food Processing." *Wisebread.* 22 MAR 2007. Web. 28 NOV 2010.

Moyer, Melinda. "It's Time to End the War on Salt." *Scientific American.* 8 JUL 2011. Web. 23 SEP 2011.

Nestle, Marion. *Safe Food: The Politics of Food Safety* (London: University of California Press 2010).

Nestle, Marion. *What To Eat* (New York: North Point Press, 2006).

Nienhiser, Jill C. "How to Avoid Genetically Modified Foods." *Westonaprice.* Spring 2008. Web. NOV 2010.

Non-GMO Project. "GMO Facts." *Nongmoproject.* Web. 17 JUNE 2012.

NPR. "America's Future Farmers Already Dropping Away." *Npr.* 27 FEB 2011. Web. 22 MAY 2012.

Organic.org. "What Does "Organic" Mean?" *Organic.* Web. 23 JUNE 2012.

Organisation for Economic Co-operation and Development (OECD). "Society at a Glance 2011 – OECD Social Indicators." *OECD.* Web. 11 May 2012.

Pollan, Michael. "Farmer in Chief." *Nytimes.* 9 OCT 2008. Web. 7 JULY 2012.

Pollan, Michael. *In Defense of Food* (England: Penguin, 2008).

Pollan, Michael. *Omnivore's Dilemma* (England: Penguin, 2007).

PR Newswire. "National Survey Reveal Disconnect Between Americans and their Food." *Prnewswire.* 22 Sept 2011. Web. 19 MAY 2012.

Prache, S. et al. "Traceability of animal feeding diet in the meat and milk of small ruminants." *Small Ruminant Research* 59.2 (2005): 157-168.

Price, Weston A. *Nutrition and Physical Degeneration* (Price-Pottenger Nutrition Foundation, 2009).

Purvis, Margarette. "Beyond the Grocery Store...Teaching Children Where Their Food Comes From." *Huffingtonpost.* 1 NOV 2011. Web. 19 MAY 2012.

Risher, Brittany. "Milk, Minus the Cow." *Womenshealthmag.* 29 AUG 2011. Web. 24 SEP 2011.

Rodale, Maria. *Organic Manifesto: How Organic Food Can Heal Our Planet, Feed the World and Keep Us Safe* (New York: Rodale Inc., 2010).

Ronald, Pamela. "Genetically Engineered Crops – What, How and Why." *Scientificamerican.* 11 AUG 2011. Web. 29 MARCH 2012.

Savage, Jessica H., et al. "The natural history of soy allergy" *The Journal of Allergy and Clinical Immunology* 125.3 (2010): 683-686.

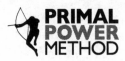

Saenz, Roberto, et al. "Confined animal feeding operations as amplifiers of influenza". *Vector-Borne and Zoonotic Diseases* 6.4 (2006): 338-346.

Salatin, Joel. *Folks This Ain't Normal* (New York: Hachette Book Group, 2011).

Schlosser, Eric. *Food, Inc.* (New York: PublicAffairs, 2009).

Schmidt, Michael. " Campaign for Real Milk." *Wise Traditions.* 11.3 (2010): 85-86.

Science Daily. "Monoculture." *Sciencedaily.* Web. 22 MAY 2012.

Shomon, Mary. "Conjugated Linoleic Acid (CLA) Supplements May Speed Weight Loss." *About.* 3 DEC 2003. Web. 14 JULY 2012.

Stanhill, G. "The comparative productivity of organic agriculture." *Agriculture, Ecosystems and Environment* 30.1 (1990): 1-26.

Staples, Todd. "Agriculture Commissioner Todd Staples says that Americans spend less of their disposable income on food than individuals in Mexico, China and Russia." *Politifact.* 29 DEC 2010. Web. 8 MAY 2012.

"Soybean Subsidies in the United States Totaled $22.8 Billion from 1995 – 2009." *Farmewg.* Web. 15 NOV 2010.

Stockholm Convention on Persistent Organic Pollutants Treaty 2004.

St-Onge, Marie-Pierre, et al. "Supplementation with Soy-Protein–Rich Foods Does Not Enhance Weight Loss." *Journal of the American Dietetic Association* 107.3 (2007): 500-505).

Sustainable Table. "Pesticides." *Sustainabletable.* Web. 7 JULY 2012.

Teng, P, et al. "Systems of plant protection." *Ciba Foundation Symposium* 177 (1993): 116-132.

The Guardian. "The 59 Ingredients in a Fast Food Strawberry Milkshake." *Guardian.* 23 APRIL 2006. Web. 11 MAY 2012.

Tran, Wendy. "Sea Salt vs. Common Table Salt." *Holistichealthlibrary.* 5 MAY 2008. Web. 7 NOV 2010.

Urban, Shilo. "What's in Fast Food Chicken? (Hint: It's NOT Chicken)." *OrganicAuthority.com.* Web. 13 SEP 2011.

Welsh, Rick. "The Economics of Organic Grain and Soybean Production in the Midwestern Untied States." *Henry A. Wallace Institute for Alternative Agriculture* (1999).

"What are Soybeans?" *Soya.* Web. 15 NOV 2010.

"What is Soy Protein?" *Soya.* Web. 15 NOV 2010.

"What is Sustainable Agriculture." *Sustainabletable.* Web. 26 OCT 2011.

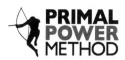

United States Department of Agriculture. "Agriculture Deputy Secretary Merrigan Announces Assistance to Help New Crop of Farmers and Ranchers." *Nifa.usda*. 20 SEP 2011. Web. 22 MAY 2012.

United States Department of Agriculture. "Bovine Spongiform Encephalopathy (BSE)." *Usda*. 2 MAY 2012. Web. 30 JUNE 2012.

United States Department of Agriculture. "Community Supported Agriculture." *Usda*. Web. 18 JULY 2012.

United States Department of Agriculture. "Food Labeling: Meat and Poultry Labeling Terms." *Fsis.usda*. 12 APRIL 2011. Web. 23 JUNE 2012.

United States Department of Agriculture. "Grading, Certification and Verification: Grass Fed Marketing Claim Standards." *Ams.usda*. 16 OCT 2007. Web. 23 June 2012.

United States Department of Agriculture. "Organic Labeling and Marketing Information." *Ams.usda*. APRIL 2008. Web. 22 MAY 2012.

United States Department of Agriculture. "Q&A on Bovine Spongiform Encephalopathy (BSE)." *Usda*. Web. June 2012.

United States Department of Agriculture. "The National List of Allowed and Prohibited Substances." *Ams.usda*. Web. 28 MAY 2012.

United States Department of Agriculture. "U.S. Beef and Cattle Industry: Background Statistics and Information." *Ers.usda*. 25 APRIL 2012. Web. 16 JUNE 2012.

United States Department of Agriculture. "U.S. Soybean Industry: Background Statistics and Information." *Usda*. Web. 15 NOV 2010.

United States Department of Agriculture Economic Research Service. "Food CPI and Expenditures: Table 7." *Usda*. 13 July 2011. Web. 11 May 2012.

United States Environmental Protection Agency. "Biopesticides." *Agriculture*. Web. 23 JAN 2014.

United States Environmental Protection Agency. "About Pesticides." *Epa*. 9 MAY 2012. Web. 7 JULY 2012.

United States Environmental Protection Agency. "Pesticides Industry Sales and Usage: 2006 and 2007 Market Estimates." January 2011.

United States Food and Drug Administration. "FDA 101: Animal Feed." *Fda*. 8 DEC 2011. Web. 30 JUNE 2012.

Yale News. "Fast Food Restaurants Dish Up Unhealthy Marketing to Youth; Researchers Release Unprecedented Report if Fast Food Nutrition and Marketing. *Yale*. 8 NOV 2010. Web. 12 MAY 2012.

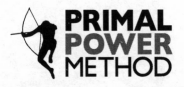

www.primalpowermethod.com

Made in the USA
Middletown, DE
23 July 2015